Bag Lady

or

Powerhouse?

A Roadmap for
Midlife (Boomer) Women

by Lillian Zimmerman

Baglady or Powerhouse?

A Roadmap for Midlife

(Boomer) Women

© 2009 Lillian Zimmerman

Library and Archives Canada
Cataloging in Publication

Zimmerman, Lillian Baglady or
powerhouse? : a roadmap for mid-life
(boomer) women / Lillian Zimmerman.

Includes index.
ISBN 978-1-55059-364-8

1. Middle-aged women--Psychology.
2. Middle-aged women--Attitudes.
3. Middle-aged women--Conduct of
life. 4. Baby boom generation. I. Title.

HQ1059.4.Z56 2009 305.244'2
C2009-900529-8

We recognize the support of the
Government of Canada through the
Book Publishing Industry Development
Pro-gram (BPIDP) for our publishing
program. We also acknowledge the
support of the Alberta Foundation for
the Arts for our publishing program.

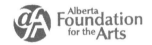

SAN 113-0234
ISBN 978-1-55059-361-7
Printed in Canada
Cover Design by James Dangerous

Detselig Enterprises
210-1220 Kensington Rd NW Calgary, AB T2N 3P5
www.temerondetselig.com p. 403-283-0900 f. 403-283-6947

To my intergenerational family, always loving and always there, my thanks.

My late parents, Ettie *and* Joseph

My daughters, Nita *and* Merle

My grandkids, in order of appearance:
Adam J., C.J., Kelsey, *and* Sean

"Look for the truth exactly on the spot where you stand." — *Buddhist saying*

Table of Contents

INTRODUCTION 11

PROLOGUE: SETTING THE STAGE 15

References 27

Chapter One

AGE, AGING, AND AGEISM:
WHERE DO WOMEN FIT IN? 29

Born Yesterday 33

*Sticks and Stones will Break My Bones
but Names will Never Hurt Me.* 37

TV or NOT TV 43

Greetings! 53

Now You See Her, Now You Don't 57

Is the Tide Turning? 65

Things You Can Do As
A Boomer Woman Change Agent 71

References 73

Chapter Two

THE PETER PAN PRINCIPLE:
MEGA-BEAUTY INDUSTRIES 81
The Anti-Aging Pressure Cookers 83
That was then, This is now 86
Early to Bed, Early to Rise –
Advertise, Advertise, Advertise 90
Never too Early to Learn 95
Marking Ourselves Down 102
The Cutting Edge 105

Things You Can Do As
A Boomer Woman Change Agent 117

References 119

Chapter Three

WHERE'S THE REST OF MY EYEBROW?
CHANGING HEALTH AND HEALTHY CHANGE 127
Historical and Hysterical 131
The Aging Enterprise 134
From Menopause to Menopower 141
Regular or Lite? 146
Illness, Wellness and Fitness 156
Women and Disability: A Slow Dance 159

Gender Benders   164

Vital Signs   170

Things You Can Do As
A Boomer Woman Change Agent   181

References   185

Chapter Four

WOMEN, WORK, AND RETIREMENT: THE WORK
BONE'S CONNECTED TO THE WAGE BONE . . .   195

*The Work Bone's Connected to
the Wage Bone*   197

*The Wage Bone's Connected to
the Caregiving Bone*   210

*The Caregiving Bone's Connected to
the Pension Bone*   221

What's Wrong With This Picture? A Critique   226

*The Pension Bone's Connected to
the Retirement Bone*   233

*To Retire or Not to Retire (and when),
That is the Question*   235

The End of Retirement?   237

Bismarck Meets the Boomers   239

*We're Mad as Hell and
Not Going to Take it Any More*   242

Things You Can Do As A Boomer Woman
Change Agent: 247

References 249

Chapter Five

THE NEW GRANDPARENTING:
MORE THAN JUST DOTING 259
Grandma, What Big Roles you Have! 264
A Kodak Moment:
Snapshots of Canadian Grandparenthood 267
Ages and Stages 269
Meanings and Values 272
Gender and Grandparenting: A Unisex Future? 274
Generationing: Adult Grandchildren 279
Case History 283
Passing it Forward: Part 1 285
Passing it Forward: Part 2 291
Gazing into a Crystal Ball:
Twenty-five Years into the Future 299

Things You Can Do As
A Boomer Woman Change Agent 300

References 302

Chapter Six

A Woman's Best Friend Is . . .   309
Smashing Some Myths   311
From Negative to Positive   313
Infrastructures, or,
How Things are Held Together   315
Buffer Zones   318
Mother/Daughter Bonds   322
Companionship   323
Cohesion   324
Conflict   325
Shock Absorbers   326
Widowhood – Not Always,
but Occasionally Merry   330
Older Lesbians and Friendship   336
Case History   340
Sisterhood is Powerful   342

Things You Can Do As
A Boomer Woman Change Agent   350

References   353

Chapter Seven

FROM RAGING HORMONES TO RAGING GRANNIES   359
Will she or won't she?   362
Setting the Table for the Twenty-First Century   370
And Now for Something Completely Different,
    or the Full Monty   375
Three Rs: Resenting,
    Resisting and Reconstructing   376
"Here's Looking at You, Kid"   388
Back to the Future (or the Beginning, or . . .)   395

References   405

Endnote   409

Appendices

APPENDIX 1: Compassionate Care   411
APPENDIX 2: The Canada Pension System   411

Index   419

Acknowledgements   425

About the Author   427

Introduction

To say that the 21st Century will be the Century of Boomer Women stands in contrast to the many ways in which the present generation of older women is ignored at best, and invisible at worst. Such a prediction can be made for reasons which this book, *Baglady or Powerhouse: A Roadmap for Midlife (Boomer) Women,* examines; and which, as the title indicates, also suggests that opportunities for midlife boomer women (those born between 1946 and 1964) to become powerhouses are within their grasp. Some already are; the majority are not. Boomer Women stand on the threshold of turning around the many psychological, cultural, and financial ways in which society currently creates barriers to their later life fulfillment. Uppermost among these are the real concerns and valid doubts many have about their ability to attain the financial security to which the frightening term "baglady" applies.

Among the reasons for making such an in-your-face prediction is that, given population aging, for the first time in Canadian history, boomer women will be the significant majority. In addition, they are "economic women" because – and also for the first time in Canadian history – boomer women will have spent the most of their adult lives in the paid work force. They are better educated, have more knowledge, and are more health conscious than their mothers or grandmothers. They seek more equality in the workforce, they engage in longer periods of study and training, and some are advancing in professions previously occupied solely by males. Many are divorced, single by choice, marrying and having children later than their mothers did; most no longer interrupt their work to attend to children to the same degree their mothers did. Numbers live openly with same sex partners.

So what's the problem?

Not all boomer women are experiencing such achievement equally. There are differences in what they earn compared to men, differences in the jobs they have and the pensions they will receive – that is, if they will get any pensions at all – and differences in the unpaid work they do. Midlife boomer and older women are the majority of family caregivers to both young and old, work that is unpaid. These are among the circumstances which lessen their chances of sailing into a golden retirement sunset.

Boomer women also exist in a popular culture that is inebriated with its worship of youth, by being and staying young, by which midlife and older women are swept aside. This includes being caricatured and made subjects of hateful, witchlike caricatures, plus idiotic "little old lady" jokes, as well as language that freely refers to older women as "old bags" or "cows". They are called "dear" or "young lady" by total strangers one third their age, and talked to loudly and slowly as though they have lost their marbles. These and other common practices distort the reality and richness of many midlife and older women's lives, and the reality of how enjoyable, productive and energetic their later lives are. Instead, such negativities fill young girls and women with distorted images, making many dread the prospect of becoming an older woman. This has to change.

It is a goal of *Baglady or Powerhouse?* to start making readers angry at the many ways they are regarded and disregarded, and to offer encouragement and motivation to make changes for both their own, their daughters or granddaughter's sakes.

My qualifications for writing this book are that I, as an older Canadian woman, have "been there," and have experienced most of the anomalies I have just outlined. I have been widowed, and raised two boomer daughters as a single parent, and now am a single grandparent. I worked at jobs which were below my capacities, earned less than I deserved, and didn't get a post-secondary education until I was (almost) a midlife woman myself. As a professional, I have worked in academic settings as an adult educator, now more popularly called lifelong learning. Throughout those years, my major motivation was always been to communicate issues that concerned women: the changing lives, the changing economic, social and cultural circumstances which affected them, the gains they made and those they have not made. It is this background which has motivated me to examine what I feel lies ahead for midlife boomer women as they traverse their personal roadmaps.

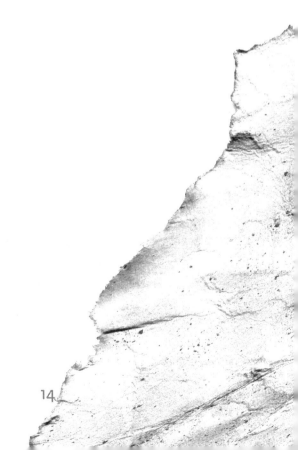

Prologue:

Setting the Stage

Population aging is one of the major developments of the 20th and 21st centuries, occurring not only in major western industrialized nations but also in the Third World. By now, many Canadians are tired of hearing what has become a mantra: that in Canada, 13% of the population is now over sixty-five, and by 2031 that figure will have doubled, to almost 25%. Life expectancy in Canada is 82.6 years for women, and 77.8 years for men.

Women over sixty-five are the fastest growing group of Canadians, and those aged eighty-five and over are aging the most rapidly.[1]

In fact, longevity makes it possible for four or even five generations of one family to live in the same time space, that is, to be alive at the same time. Midlife and older women and men are co-existing with daughters, sons, daughters-in-law and sons-in-law, even granddaughters, grandsons and their partners and children and, in some instances, their great-grandchildren. There is much to be learned from the complex ways in which generations, most certainly midlife boomer women, are currently interacting and intertwining: both inter- and intragenerationally.

The breaking news is good. These momentous demographic changes are affecting women's lives in important ways. For one thing, boomer women, especially as they age, will become the majority. Their lives are already far different than those lived by their mothers and grandmothers, many of the changes definitely for the better. They include more education, higher participation in the paid work force, doing work that was traditionally for men only, and a wider range of choices with regard to marriage, having children, and not interrupting work as long to stay home and look after younger children. Also, boomers are "wired" technologically, and because of computers, e-mails, faxes, ipods, blackberries, cell phones and text-messaging, their lives are on fast forward.

But there are other things that are important for boomer women to know because, in fact, the Canadian boomer generation – most especially the women – is one of the most unique in history. Let's look at why this is so.

The late Betty Friedan's landmark 1963 book, *The Feminine Mystique*, is credited with starting the women's movement of the 1960s, but in 1993 she wrote another book, *The Fountain of Age*, that is not nearly as well known, but contains more valuable insights for the 21st century.[2] One of Friedan's major points is her assertion that, because people are living longer, boomer women (and to a lesser degree men, since they don't live as long) are – in her words – "biological pioneers." What she means is that by living longer, mid-life boomer women are occupying a stage of life that barely existed before. They are entering a new area where there are few signposts or other markers to guide them. This can be interpreted to mean that the occupants of this new social stage, the midlife boomer women, will be able to create and establish new ways of living their lives. The renowned American gerontologist Robert Butler has called this "the longevity revolution," a movement that he feels will be as powerful as any of the great economic and social movements of the past thirty years, including the women's movement.[3]

Flowing from this – the recognition of a new social stage of life which boomer women and men occupy – is the possibility for further development. What I mean by this is the idea that we see each stage of life as developing into the next one. An infant will develop into a baby, who will then proceed to be a toddler, move along to be a young child, and then grow into a teenager. The teenager becomes an adult, then enters middle age, which in turn develops into old age. Period. And at present that's where the prospect of development stops-at the socially, not biologically, designated age of sixty-five. But on average, women still have twenty or thirty more years of life ahead in which to experience, grow and develop. However, this new developmental stage of life is rarely considered as such.

If fact, sixty-five has become the societal marker of the beginning of decline, though sometimes this marker has been set even earlier for women. Midlife women, often aged well below sixty-five, can find it difficult to get jobs, or jobs that they want.

But is it necessarily true that sixty-five means the beginning of decline? Absolutely not. And this is what social analyst Margaret Morganroth Gullette writes about so convincingly in her book *Declining to Decline*.[4] What she means by her title and what is so important for midlife boomer women to realize is that we are aged more by culture than by biology. The essence of this idea is that women learn to be old because of the way they are portrayed in popular culture. Older women are stereotyped and shown as anything but attractive by a youth-iconized popular culture that includes TV, movies, the media, greeting cards, language and attitudes. Another writer, Margaret Cruikshank, makes clear in her book *Learning to be Old* that "aging . . . is shaped more by culture than by biology, more by beliefs, customs and traditions than by bodily changes."[5] This can have debilitating consequences for women because they come to fear growing older when, in fact, their later lives – midlife and forward – can be among the most fulfilling and enjoyable times, a stage of life which can be – and is, in fact – full of vitality. However, we rarely hear this expressed, and midlife boomer women need to hear it.

Two questions need to be considered here. The first is: who and what are the boomers and what makes them such a unique generation? Both timing and numbers are the qualities and quantities that shaped their uniqueness. Canadian boomers were born approximately between 1946 and 1964. This "boomer bulge" began just after the end of World War II when soldiers returned from the battles of Europe and Japan and women workers like "Rosie the Riveter" were "relieved" of their jobs to make work available to the returning armed forces. Undoubtedly, lost time and long separations motivated an extraordinary amount of activity in the bedrooms of the nation (with apologies to Pierre Elliott Trudeau).

Or perhaps the lack of such distractions as television, videos, video games, computers and the internet contributed to the increased birthrate because whatever the reasons, the results were remarkable. The startling fact is that, second to the United States, Canada has the largest boomer population anywhere. There are an estimated nine million of them, and they are almost evenly divided by gender, meaning there will be some four and a half million Canadian boomer women reaching formal retirement age between 2011 and 2029. Some of the leading edge boomers, having turned 60 in 2006, have already retired.

The second questions is: why is my book *only* about women? It most certainly is not a hate-men exercise, but instead concerns the social, economic, cultural and psychological underpinnings that, as several social observers have stated, make aging a woman's issue.[6]

This is also referred to as the social construction of women's aging. These are socio-economic facts: women earn 71% of what men earn in their lifetimes; almost 28% of women work only part-time, due primarily to family responsibilities; women live longer than men; they remarry at lower rates than men; they are the majority of caregivers, not only of children but increasingly of aging elders; they have fewer pensions and receive lesser benefits than men. The number of widows exceeds that of widowers, and widow's incomes generally decline as most certainly divorced women's incomes do.

Because of a combination of all or some of these variables, many older women are poorer than older men in Canada. In fact, Statistics Canada reported that in 2006, the percentage of unattached women aged sixty-five and over in low income was 37.2% before tax, contrasted to 28.9% of men in the same category. The incomes of these unattached men and women has decreased significantly in recent years, still over 37% of unattached older women living at or below the poverty line is unacceptable.[7]

There is one other perspective about boomers that deserves attention, that being the popular belief that boomers have changed each stage of life as they occupied it, frequently referred to as the "me generation." In fact, a recent book by Leonard Steinhorn, *The Greater Generation*, goes to the extreme – in my assessment – of claiming that boomers are the greatest generation that has ever lived, transforming major aspects of American society completely.[8] According to this theory, now that the leading edge of the boomer generation has reached age 60, we can expect that they will transform our notions about aging as well. To what degree are these assertions accurate, to what degree are they popular myth, and how relevant are they for midlife boomer women?

There are no easy answers. In fact, even a cursory look reveals that boomers' lives – especially boomer women's lives – contain many contradictions. Paul Hodge of Harvard University recognizes many of the unique financial hurdles that boomer women face, including the number of years in the workforce, caregiving responsibilities, lower earnings and longevity.[9] And Gail Marks Jarvis addressed women's issues in an article with the headline "Investment anxiety spurs bag-lady fear," citing women's fears about their financial futures.[10]

These are American citations, but a comprehensive special section of the *Globe and Mail* called "Boom Baby Boom" recently had various authors look at the massive effect boomers have had this past half-century, its values, culture and commerce.[11] One of the important things that the study points out are the differences among those we call boomers. The authors separate boomer cohorts into three age groups, describing how the older cohorts, now sixty, got jobs and bought homes before prices skyrocketed. This cohort reaped benefits, but the next, the fifty-year aged cohorts, the biggest boomer bulge, had to fight to get ahead, among other things because of their large numbers and greater competition.

The third group, the youngest boomers, claim they had the toughest time, living in the shadows of their older counterparts, who blocked their career paths and inflated real estate prices. They worry about paying for pensions and Medicare. This is a valuable analysis making clear as it does that Canadian "boomers" are not all the same – in fact there is a twenty-year spread encompassing different attitudes and concerns. The study features a Strategic Counsel poll, describing Canadian boomers as a "mess of contradictions." It states: "You [boomers] are either the most optimistic generation ever to walk the earth or the most self-deluded."[12] The contradictions range from the "me" generation, interested in immediate gratification, to those more affected by the great social currents that "washed across the decades" – feminism, the sexual revolution, war, the environment fitness and religion. Despite boomers' general optimism, the poll showed them to be a stressed generation, struggling to balance the needs of their parents and their children while worrying about their retirement.

Whether boomer women will transform age as we know it, considering the many contradictions of the large boomer cohorts, remains to be seen, but I feel it is within their grasp to level the playing fields .

In writing *Baglady or Powerhouse*, I make no claim to objectivity. *Au contraire.* My purpose is to highlight what I perceive as the serious neglect of the many ways in which aging has become a woman's issue. I say this as an older woman, because I believe that there is a bridge between the current generation of older women and the upcoming mid-life boomer women because "we" (older women) have been there, have stories to tell about the barriers we have faced, some of which we overcame though others are still there for midlife boomers albeit in different terms. How we accomplished this is important for boomer women to know. Further, there is a great deal of excellent academic literature about mid-life women in journal articles, books, research and analyses of women's lives, not easily accessed by a general audience of boomer women. I want to make some of this available to mid-life women because much of the writing contains very valuable information and ideas concerning them.

In addition I refer to many forms of popular culture such as TV, movies, language, newspapers and the internet. Further, because I feel that if one wants to know what older and midlife women think about their experiences, the things that shaped their lives and other significant events over their lifecourses then speaking to them directly is the way to go. To this end, I organized six focus groups of women aged fifty-five and older, structuring the groups around the topics my book discusses, and I have sprinkled their comments throughout it. I have also interviewed many mid-life boomer women whose comments are similarly cited, in addition to a number of case histories.

My book is not so much a guide as it is a compass. It will not show anyone how to become a sexual hottie at age fifty, nor what stock to invest in to assure financial independence in later years. Instead, it asks the reader to invest in herself. It points in the direction of the new territory which midlife boomer women are occupying, the developmental possibilities therein, and outlines the terrain which they will navigate. It is time – in fact, well past the time – to make changes so that women do not reach their later lives without sufficient resources or the threat of insufficient resources. I have a strong resentment when I read how many older Canadian women, who have done everything expected of them, continue to struggle in their later lives. This is simply unacceptable. I want boomer women not only to resent it but to find ways to turn things around.

Some months ago I was in line at a hosiery counter in a major department store behind an older woman, her yellowish-white hair tied in a knot at the nape of her neck. She was anything but fashionable in her dark green, rather shabby sweater and un-matching skirt. While she was speaking to the staff woman behind the counter, a younger woman came charging in and, breathlessly ignoring the queue, spoke directly to the sales person, who then left the counter to assist the young woman with whatever she needed so urgently. I remarked to the older woman in front of me that this interruption was uncalled for. She turned, looked at me rather sadly, and said, "That's all right. I'm used to being ignored." While I don't know the personal details of her life, I have a pretty good idea about the life she lived, probably doing all the things expected of her, and how she came to feel the way she did now that she was older.

Although the ad says, "You've come a long way, baby," there is still a long way to go before significant numbers of mid-life boomer women will sail into a financially and otherwise more secure golden sunset in their later years. My message is: Go for it.

References

1. Statistics Canada, The Daily, Dec. 20, 2006. *Women in Canada: A Gender Based Statistical Report* (5th Ed., Cat.no. 89-503-XPE, 2006), 265-267.

2. Betty Friedan, *The Fountain of Age* (New York: Simon and Schuster, 1993), 155.

3. Robert N. Butler, *personal communication*, 2006.

4. Margaret Morganroth Gullette, *Declining to Decline: Cultural Combat and the Politics of Midlife* (Charlottesville and London: University Press of Virginia, 1997).

5. Margaret Cruikshank, *Learning to be Old: Gender, Culture, and Aging* (Lanham: Rowan & Littlefield Publishers Inc, 2003).

6. Sharon McIrvine, Abu-Laben, and Susan A. McDaniel, "Beauty, Status, and Aging" in *Feminist Issues: Race, Class and Sexuality*, 4th Ed., ed. Nancy Mandell (Toronto, ON: Pearson Education Centre, 2004).

7. Statistics Canada, Table *Persons in low income before tax, by prevalence in percent*. <http:www40.statcan.ca/101.cst01/famil41a.> Retrieved 6/5/2008. Note: Canada does not have an official poverty line. The Low-Income Cutoffs (LIC0) is used to convey those in "straitened

circumstances." See also Statistics Canada Annual *Income in Canada*. Cat.no. 750202-XIE (2006). Also, the National Council of Welfare *Poverty Statistics 2004* for poverty by age and sex. See also Canadian Association of Social Workers (CASW) "Financial Security for Women Seniors in Canada" (2007).

8. Leonard Steinhorn, *The Greater Generation: In Defense of the Baby Boom Legacy* (New York: Thomas Dunne Books, St.Martin's Press, 2006).

9. Paul Hodge, *One Expert's Opinion: Aging Population Will Transform Society*, < http://www.genpolicy.com/articles/hodge_generation_policy_022304.html> (accessed September 7, 2006).

10. Gail Marks Jarvis, "Investment Anxiety spurs bag-lady-fears," Chicago Tribune, September 3, 2006 <http://archives.chicagotribune.com/2006/s/sep/03/business/chi-0609030324sep.03> (accessed September 6, 2006).

11. "Boom Baby Boom," *Globe and Mail*, Section F, June 24, 2006.

12. Ibid: F, 15.

Chapter One

Age, Aging and Ageism:
Where do Women Fit in?

"We are all recovering ageists."
    — Margaret Gullette

"Who would you rather be, Tina Turner or Whistler's Mother?" ran a newspaper headline describing one of the sessions at the 2001 International Association of Gerontology's Congress. Of course, most mid-life women wouldn't hesitate to choose Tina Turner – the talented, energetic, sixty-something entertainer – as a model for their roadmap. And they would be right since the majority of mid-life boomer women and most older women today are healthy, full of vitality, productive and hardly ready to sit passively in a rocking chair.

One of the problems, however, is that the world we live in, as represented by our popular culture, has yet to recognize this changed reality. In fact, not too many boomer women look forward with much enthusiasm to getting older. Given the exposure boomer women have had to a wide range of media and being bombarded by advertising that is mostly negative towards older women, small wonder their fantasies about growing older fill them with fear. This is not to say that today's older generation of women, who in their youth had mainly the radio to bring the world to them, were held in higher esteem in the 1930s and `40s or, for that matter, throughout earlier history. A look at the language we use about older women makes this clear.

But the advent of television in the 1950s, when the leading cohort of mid-life boomer women were young children, made them the first generation to grow up with it. Indeed, it was the proliferation of television and a growing corporate structure pursuing a new market niche, that of selling to the young, that increased the exponential influence of TV advertising, while at the same time advertising was increasing in the print media. First they concentrated on selling through the parents, then as this new generation aged, they sold directly to teenagers, which helped to establish a culture of youth. (More recently they began skipping the first step and selling directly to toddlers.) Looking young, they said, means looking good. Thus, being an older women gets short shrift, and this is really too bad because women's later years can be among the richest of their lives, and hold the potential to get richer.

However, you wouldn't know this by growing up and living in today's (and yesterday's) popular culture because television, movies, language and jokes constantly teach us otherwise. This has become a culture in which youth is the standard by which everyone is judged. While the terms "sexism" and "racism" have long been part of our cultural understanding, "ageism" is just beginning to be recognized as a social problem. The word attributed to an American gerontologist, Robert Butler, simply means the dislike of or discrimination against older people because of their age. Ageism is now receiving a great deal of attention and long overdue study, but when it comes to studying women as they age, there's still a long way to go, baby.

Although all older people are subject to ageist beliefs, women are by far the most common targets. Older and midlife women are bombarded with negative stereotypes, images and depictions which do them much harm, influencing the less-than-positive ways they view themselves. This can result in plummeting self-esteem and damaging self-images even to the point of self-hatred, which has no place on boomer women's roadmaps.

I submitted an early draft of this chapter to a respected publisher and was told that the topic of ageism in the media, movies, TV and language is by now well-known, and I needed to say something new. I don't agree. I believe the fact that ageism continues in the 21st century in relation to women growing older is itself news and deserving of attention;

indeed, demanding attention. It continues to exert its negative influence on boomer women about growing older in a youth-besotted society.

Another dimension is the development in the past decade of the notion of 'Successful Aging'. As Calastani and Slevin assert, some feminists accept the notion of aging successfully.[1] These writers feel that this reinforces ageism. "Successful aging requires maintenance of the activities popular among the middle-agers privileged with money and leisure time." In other words, the successful aging concept targets well-to-do middle class women, ignoring class, race, and other differences. Many less affluent women have neither the money nor time to engage in fitness classes in order to remain slim and sexy (more of this in Chapter 3).

Thus we do not need to seek 'something newer' in our attempt to understand the mechanism of ageism, especially its bias against older women. Ageism not only continues, but appears in new forms. Seeking to understand this continuing dilemma is the important idea that we are aged more by culture than by biology. The cultural construction of aging, which means how society and social institutions organize the frameworks which set up standards of acceptable and non-acceptable norms, governs our social lives. A midlife woman, for example, is frowned on if she trots around in tight mini-skirts, net stockings, and stiletto heels, because this attire goes against accepted social standards. The fact is that we are aged more by culture than by biology. Yes, we all get older biologically, but the social and cultural constructions of aging mean that women are not supposed to look old, and are rejected if they do so, even though staying young forever is impossible. I talked to a boomer woman in her early fifties – a receptionist in a large credit union – who was going through menopause, which caused her face to redden at times. Her immediate superior, a male in his late twenties, took her off the reception desk and placed her at a desk somewhere out of sight, claiming that her flushed face put clients off! This incident underlines the idea behind the cultural construction of aging: that we learn to be old through the influence of various aspects of culture. In fact, *Learning to be Old* (Lantham, Rowe & Littlefield, 2003) by Margaret Cruikshank makes clear how societal pressures affect women as they age, teaching them, in effect to fear getting older.[2]

Born Yesterday

Unflattering images of older women did not just spring up in recent years, but rather have a long history from ancient Greece up to today. One expert in Grecian art described surviving depictions of recognizably older women as either comic or pitiable.[3]

Damaging depictions of older women are also expressed in folklore and fairy tales. Hansel and Gretel fall into the hands of a wicked old witch, who burns little children in an oven. And Rapunzel is imprisoned in a tower by an evil crone. Researcher Elizabeth Markson traces such misogyny or the hatred of women through a number of world societies. For example, she finds Scottish mythology is liberally strewn with references to such powerful old crones. And she cites an old Arab belief that, when each child is born, it is surrounded by one hundred angels. For every year a male lives an angel is added, but for every year a female lives an angel dies.[4] Not a very encouraging way for a girl to start life. In *The Quest for Immortality: Science at the Frontiers of Aging* (W.W. Norton, 2001), authors S. Jay Olshansky and Bruce Carnes point out that "The idea that women are responsible for aging and death is a recurring theme in history chronicled principally by men."[5] They demonstrate that this is true in myth as well. For example, "Zeus created Pandora, the first woman, who had 'charming traits' to hide her wicked nature . . . The jar that Pandora brought with her to the world was filled with evil things, including among them plagues, disease, and old age."

Although postmenopausal women were accorded a reasonably favourable status in some societies, possibly because they were beyond their reproductive years and thus no longer in competition, as it were, these societies are the exception rather than the rule. In most societies, images of witches were based on the belief that women had supernatural powers associated with fertility, and when they reached menopause, it was believed they came into possession of magical powers so strong that it affected male sexual prowess. This was clearly long before Viagra, and may have been the affliction that is now called erectile dysfunction (ED), but older women became the scapegoats, accused of being witches and burned at the stake or drowned. Well, sometimes not exactly drowned, because if she was submerged and lived, she was held to be a witch and then burned at the stake. If she did drown, then it was believed that she had not been a witch after all. Talk about a Catch-22! In any case, it was certainly one way to get rid of poor, usually single, old women: some two million of them.[7]

It would be joyful to be able to say that now, in the 21st century, we no longer disparage older women. However such is not the case. In Cruikshank's book *Learning to be Old*, she comments, "The witch craze is like a toxic waste site covered up for a long time but still emitting poisons. The hatred of old women that is its legacy is fairly well concealed in our society."[8] But not quite that "well concealed" as it turns out, according to a finding by a media watch group that is critical of the way the press disparages politically active women. This group found that when Hilary Clinton was still the

American First Lady, she was referred to as a "witch" or "witchlike" at least fifty times. Their report goes on to ponder why male political leaders are never called warlocks. When Clinton announced her candidacy to be president of the US in the 2008 election, she was referred to as a hag or harridan. As if that wasn't enough a columnist for *Rolling Stone*, though himself critical of Clinton, recognizes that she has been pilloried, portrayed variously as a lesbian, an evil socialist, and "a late middle age lived out as an unsmiling pro-military curmudgeon with a fast-rusting vagina." I rest my case regarding the idea that media ageism is by now old hat.

In addition, during Hillary Clinton's candidacy for President of the US during the 2007/2008 campaign, her treatment by the media was frequently denounced as being sexist by both feminists and other journalists concerned with women's rights . The following article is a typical example.[10]

Writing that "Clinton a constant target of sexist remarks" Edna declaimed the double standard afforded male candidates as contrasted with Clinton's. "She is judged differently than her male competitors . . . When she doesn't show emotion, she's cold. When she does, she's – what? – feminine? Soft? Uncommander-in-chief-like? . . . When she's serious, she's humorless: if she laughs, she cackles. If she attacks she's partisan . . . If she wears pantsuits, she's manly. If she shows a millimeter of cleavage, she's flirty."

Indeed, the 2008 candidacy for US President had the unintended consequence of revealing just how alive both sexism and ageism are. If Enda's examples are not enough, Clinton was the target of a group calling itself "Citizens United Not Timid" (check the capitals). There was also of a vicious cartoon showing her with splayed legs and a nutcracker with metal spikes between her thighs. Ageism with respect to older women (Clinton was 60) not only exists, but does in a manner which is egregious in the extreme.

Sticks and Stones will Break My Bones but Names will Never Hurt Me.

Contrary to what this old nursery rhyme says, names will hurt, as will words. In an article on ageism and ageist language published in *The Journal of Social Issues* in 2005, a group of respected researchers state that ageism is pervasive in our society – in the media, health care, education, the workplace, and everyday conversation. Here is part of what they say about older adults. "Societal stereotypes and ageist language inaccurately group this population, often resulting in serious consequences not only for older adults, but also to all members of society who actively participate in the social construction of aging and the physical aging process."[11] The writers go on to say that derogatory language about older adults underwrites feelings by some that such persons are a burden. Further, it can cause older people to see decline as inevitable, which in turn encourages passivity.

Close your eyes and think of what you see when you hear the phrase "older woman." Got it? All right, close them again and think of the phrase "elderly woman." In all likelihood, the image conjured up by the first phrase will differ from that conjured up by the second, in that the second will likely evoke an image of frailty. Of course, frail elderly women and men do exist, but when one constantly hears the word elderly or keeps seeing it regularly in newspapers, one forms the false picture that all elderly women are dependent and needful. And this simply is not the case.

However, it is not only the words themselves that are the problem, but also the way they are spoken. When talking to an older person, younger people – perhaps mistakenly thinking they are being helpful – sometimes slow down their speech, pick up the volume, and e-n-u-n-c-i-a-t-e v-e-r-y c-l-e-a-r-l-y. It would appear they think the person they are addressing is dimwitted, and probably hard-of-hearing to boot (interestingly, this is also precisely how ignorant people address those who do not speak their language).

Further, younger people are often patronizing and condescending when speaking to an older woman, frequently addressing her as "young lady" or referring her as "dear" although the person speaking may be less than half her age. One woman taking part in the focus groups I organized in preparation for this book reported that a younger security man at the front door of a public building held the door open for her and called her "my pet." Most of the other women in the group objected to being called "young lady," although one did say it depended on who was saying it.

Interestingly, a couple of boomer women in their late fifties whom I interviewed did not object at all to being called "young lady," feeling that it was flattering. There are likely others who feel the same. With regard to addressing older women in an unacceptable fashion, there is a heartening anecdote about the late Gerald Ford, the former US president who, it is asserted, got his come-uppance when he made the mistake of addressing the late, great Maggie Kuhn, she of Gray Panthers fame, by asking her, "What have you got to say, young lady?" She is said to have replied, "Mr. President I am not a young lady. I'm an old woman." Later she commented, "I just couldn't help reminding him that his words weren't a compliment." Of course, we rarely hear of an older male politician or corporate executive or indeed any older male being addressed as "young man." What does this tell us?

People who address mid-life and older women in such a fashion may feel that they are being complimentary, but in reality they have succumbed to the idea that older means to be in decline, both mentally and physically. One older woman with a younger female partner recalled that when she was in a store, the clerk ignored her and addressed all his remarks to the younger partner.[12] The experience led her to believe that older women are invisible. This was ageism, pure and simple. However, an older person being ignored is more common when the woman is with a male and all remarks are addressed to him – in which case, the treatment is both sexist and ageist.

A number of studies have looked at how ageism is reflected in the words used to describe older women. At De Paul University, Professor Frida Furman asked her students to describe older people. The class presented a list of adjectives that were clearly ageist, including sickly, absent-minded, lonely, inactive, useless, crabby, whiney, and ineffective. She then asked for descriptions of older women only. These are some of the words they chose: domestic, nostalgic, interfering, out of shape, bitter, overbearing, frustrated, needy, stubborn, a liability, worn-down, gaudy, wrinkled, rambling, busybody, hag, wicked, evil nag, constant complainer, meddler, gossip, crooked, shrinking, widowed, helpless, tea-drinking, arthritic, bingo-playing, liver spots.[13] It is well to remember that these were young students, probably between seventeen and nineteen, but reading these descriptions, one wonders if any of them ever had mothers, grandmothers, or older aunts. It was not difficult for this professor to surmise that "we can readily arrive at the conclusion that older people in general and older women specifically are depicted in stereotypic ways, often viciously so."[14]

Yet another source cites similarly offensive words being applied to older women, among them: biddy, crone, grimalkin, hag, little old lady, old maids, shrew, old bag, old bat, old battle axe, spinster, and witch.[15]

There are also unflattering descriptions of older men (for example, old fart, curmudgeon, crabby, cantankerous, old droopy pants, geezer, and coot), but they come nowhere near the same degree of intensity and insult as those applied to older women.

Then there are the adjectives that a writer or speaker may mistakenly consider to be expressing admiration. For example, "feisty" is often used to describe active older women, but MacDonald and Rich, in their book *Look Me in the Eye*, point out that "feisty means touchy, excitable, quarrelsome . . . [and] is the standard word . . . for an older person who says what she thinks. As you grow older, the younger person sees your strongly felt convictions or your protest against an intolerable life situation as an amusing over-reaction."[16] This attitude effectively trivializes and thus marginalizes older women's concerns: it is not what she's saying that becomes the focus so much as how she is perceived to be saying it. In effect, it erases her intent.

A male Canadian columnist referred dismissively to the endeavours of a group of older women by calling them "little permed women."

Finally, there is the demeaning language that women use with respect to themselves and to each other. Referring to one's "boobs" rather than to breasts is a common example of how women get caught up in words that basically devalue their bodies. So is calling oneself a "broad" or "little old lady" or "having a senior's moment."

In this vein, I would like to suggest that the word "senior" should itself be retired. There are two reasons to consider this.

First, with the current downsizing of social programs and concern with bottom lines, seniors are scapegoated and declared drains on public safety nets, even though this is not the case. Women, because they live longer than men, are especially targeted.

Second, the term is increasingly invalid and culturally devalued to a significant extent. It was originally used to denote a fairly high status, as contrasted, for example, with "junior." Now it is used simply to mean "old". In fact, all the current language relating to aging is obsolete and, according to a study by the Harvard School of Public Health, may actually be an impediment to change.[17]

This is an important point, suggesting as it does, that continued use of the word "senior" will slow up public recognition of the many changes taking place in the lives of midlife boomers. It also reinforces the notion of decline, failing as it does to recognize the further stages of development older boomers have just ahead of them.

In addition, now that leading edge boomers have reached the age of sixty, there is a curious overlap with the word "senior," which is now informally taken to be sixty, and in some cases fifty-five, rather than the formal, legislated age of sixty-five. Does this place sixty-plus boomers in a new category of "junior seniors"?

TV or NOT TV

The classic 1950s TV comedy series *I Love Lucy*, starring Lucille Ball, is revered for many reasons. Ball was one of the earliest female television stars, and pioneered the situation comedy, or sitcom, that is now standard TV fare. Her antics were both imaginative and funny. Sometimes her character was trying to get a job in show business; at other times she and her friend Ethel (played by Vivian Vance) attempted to raise money for shopping sprees or other activities. Few of us will forget the show where Lucy and Ethel were hired to work in a chocolate factory and wound up eating or throwing the chocolates in their caps to keep up with the speeding machine. But these antics attested to the mores of the times: women as adorable housewives, dependent on good-hearted hubbies for their finances and for permission to realize personal ambitions.

While their friendship depicted a relationship between younger (Lucy) and an older (Ethel) woman, which was in itself admirable, in fact, Ball was forty playing a twenty-nine-year-old, and Vance, who was two years younger than Ball, had to agree to wear "frumpy" clothes as befitted an "older woman."

Times have certainly changed, and TV with it, but its portrayal of mid-life boomer and older women today still leaves much to be desired. More recent series, such as *Cybill, Kate and Allie,* and *Murphy Brown* depict younger middle-aged women as being strong in their own right, though women in the official "senior" bracket are still generally portrayed as frail and addled.

Interestingly, though seldom noted, is a positive dynamic associated with older actors and characters in "soap operas" that deal with extended families and generations as they age. Early "soaps," as they are generally known, were shown during the day, and were directed at women in the home who were considered to be the chief consumers of soap by virtue of the fact that they did all the laundry (do I hear you saying that they still do?) One closet soap watcher I interviewed, herself a boomer mid-life woman, told me that *All My Children* had started in the 1970s, and that its central male and female characters have continued to age naturally with the show. For example, Ruth Warrick originated her role of Phoebe Tyler Wallingford in 1970, and played it until her death in January 2005 at the age of eighty-eight. Her last episode was aired ten days before she died. My respondent also felt that the actors in *General Hospital* have demonstrated their characters continuing to age. Furthermore, when an actor has suffered a stroke hearing loss, it appears to be the policy that this will be simply written into the script, and they will continue on in their role. It would be interesting to know the shows' reasons for doing so, as it appears to be atypical of the portrayal of older people in other television offerings.

Overall, the statistics are not good. The winter 1999 edition of *The Media Report to Women* reports that in the year 1997-98, women accounted for 39% of all characters in top-rated programs on prime time television, but that better than two-thirds or 65% of these female characters were in their twenties and thirties. This report also noted that when women worked behind the scenes as executive producers and so on, more female characters appeared. And when female writers worked on the show, female characters were given more powerful dialog.[18]

For a different take on the effects of television on a daughter of boomer parents, see the recently published Allison Klein book, *What Would Murphy Brown Do? How the Women of Prime Time Changed Our Lives* (Seal Press, 2006).

In 2002, British researchers Tim Healey and Karen Ross found that TV does not appear to be presenting images of older people that are consonant with the changed times. What they did to come to these conclusions – and what not too many others have done – is talk directly to older viewers about the images on their TV screens. The group responses included animosity towards advertising of products and services that was grossly patronizing; they specifically name stair lifts and undergarments for incontinence. They resented negative stereotyping of older people who were shown as "dependent, frail, vulnerable, poor, worthless, asexual, isolated, grumpy, behind the times, stupid, miserable, ga-ga, pathetic, and a drain on society."[19] How's that for telling it like it is?

This British research team also looked at American material on this topic and, although it found some improvement, concluded that very little has changed in recent years. It does appear that some changes are being felt about television with regard to diversity in women's roles. A 2007 report found that "From *Xena: Warrior Princess* to *Judging Amy*, television shows are redefining women in dramatic roles by telling diverse stories about their lives," according to a US academic. The report continues "The number of female-centred dramas jumped to 14 in 1985-1994, up from eight shows during 1975-1984. In 1995-2005, the number jumped to about 37 shows, peaking in 2000 as television executives and advertisers saw the value of developing strategies to target the female audience."[20]

A 2004 study concerning the portrayal of older people in prime time German television series found overall that older aged people were under-represented, excessively homogeneous and stereotypes.[21] This gendered study found among other variables, that men were shown to get more help with women giving more help; that men were also shown more positively as 'winners' and older people were portrayed more positively than was the case in real life. The authors felt this has negative effects for older viewers regarding their self-esteem, and also influences how younger watchers come to view older people.

There was one finding which in the author's words were "especially remarkable" in the prime-time series they studied: The majority, all over sixty years of age, were in the work force. Older women were no longer shown as caring housewives and grandmothers, as had been the case in the 80s and 90s, but as working women. However, the work men did was seen to be of high status, whereas the work women did was shown as unskilled. This is an important finding as these prime time TV series recognized such major demographic shifts as older women now being in the workforce.

TV and advertising are, of course, inseparable, and many TV ads directed toward older women leave one with a distinct impression that all older women are in decline. For example, one recent ad shows people getting off a bus and being asked where they are going. When a white-haired older woman gets off, she responds in a silly voice, "I'm going to see my boyfriend." The dialog put into these actors' mouths manages to be both ageist and sexist, with the mocking subtext clearly being that older women are not sexual beings and, if they are, they shouldn't be. The writers, probably young males, were not aiming at normalcy, but rather at getting attention by depicting an older woman's sexual foolishness.

Another TV ad that appears to be full of promise shows three older men reacting when an attractive older woman comes into the room. Their eyes pop out and, as the camera focuses on her bosom, one of them asks, "Are those real?" Then the shot moves up to her teeth. It is dentures, of course, that are being pitched, but a full bosom is featured in order to get the viewer's attention – unless some women carry their dentures in their bras. Again, this ad manages to be both sexist and ageist.

A number of older women I talked to expressed their distaste for "Depends" advertising, as well as for other products they felt were best discussed in a doctor's office. Incontinence is certainly what some older women do experience, but it is far from inevitable. One of my women informants felt that "across the board, the commercials show young and beautiful people advertising products. They should show older women, too." And a comment from a boomer woman I talked to was to the effect that "older men [on television] get to look better with age, but older women don't." An exception to these observations occurs when the advertiser is selling expensive retirement homes or financial products. Then the couples (and they usually are couples) are radiant, bursting with good health and energy, their gray hair fairly sparkling in the sunlight as they bound off towards the tennis courts. No adult diapers here! But what these ads actually do, although this is not their intent, is make the point that wealth and health go together. An article on advertisers in the Canadian national newspaper *The Globe and Mail* claimed that "to people over fifty advertising often looks like a vast commercial sea spilled forth by the fountain of youth . . . the actors all look like they're in high school. And their dialog is punctuated with 'like' or 'whatever'."[22]

While there can be arguments over whether there is a cause and effect relationship between televised or print images and attitudes towards older people, there is general agreement in published research about the relative absence of older characters in both programming and advertising. However, one study in the United States found that advertisers are beginning to be more cognizant of the consumer powers of graying boomers. And a Yale University epidemiologist testified to a Special Senate Committee on Aging that "although the prevalence of negative images of aging is not entirely due to the media and marketing, they seem to be the sources that are the most pervasive, identifiable, systematic and profit driven. Extolling youth while demeaning the old helps to generate images that . . . may have devastating consequences."[23]

And – we can add – contributes to the whole culture of learning to be old. By emphasizing decline, such depictions fail to recognize that midlife boomer women are in the process of "becoming," not declining.

I did find one hopeful source of representations of people over fifty. In an examination of the advocacy magazine *Modern Maturity* that was published in the *Journal of Applied Gerontology*, the investigators found that, while recent research suggests nothing much has changed in general advertising, the publishers of this magazine have a policy of screening for advertisements that they consider to be negative and ageist. Over the years, this policy has proven successful and images of both gender and age have come close to being reasonable. More of this type of screening would be helpful.[24]

Where are our positive and joyful images of older women? This is the question asked by Janice Pearson, a mid-life woman and expert on women's health, who goes on to ask how midlife and older women can feel comfortable about aging in a society where youth and beauty are prized, and the older woman becomes invisible and less sexual.[25] This is an important question, her point being that negative depictions of middle-aged women hardly encourage them to feel enthusiastic about their aging.

Another strong point is made by researchers Andrea Press and Terry Strathman, who found that even when alterations have been made in television images, they have not always paralleled societal shifts, particularly with regards to women.[26] Writing about representations of work, family, and social class in prime time television images of women, they point out that popular television narratives minimize the problems of contemporary American women, as they attempt to "carve out new identities for themselves during rapidly changing social realities and expectations."[27] These writers cite a National Commission on Working Women, which found that current television portrayals of women fail to represent not only poorer single mothers, but also the pressures on women who are balancing work with family, finding child care, stretching family budgets, and so on.

Given the current lives of Canadian women, with 76% of women between forty-five and fifty-four, and 46% of women aged fifty-five and sixty-four in the paid workforce, instead of *Desperate Housewives* it would be far more realistic to present a series called

Desperate Jugglers: Women Managing Home and Work; this would represent the realities of working women's constant multi-tasking.[28]

Of course, we watch TV to be entertained, but given television's strong influence in shaping our attitudes and views, a bit more realism about boomer women's lives certainly wouldn't hurt.

Representation of needed image change portraying current mid life women could be the role Candace Bergen played in *Boston Legal*. Her role depicts her as a natural, assertive working midlife women in the real world.

It may be that TV is showcasing more and more interesting women, such as Kyra Sedgewick as Deputy Police Chief Brenda Johnson on *The Closer*, Judy Davis playing Nancy Reagan in *The Reagans,* and Helen Mirren as Detective Chief Inspector Jane Tennison in *Prime Suspect*, among others.

While, and thankfully, gains have been made with regard to depictions of lesbian women – Ellen DeGeneres and Rosie O'Donnell, for example – depictions of older lesbian women are few and far between. Publicity regarding the series *The L Word* features a photo of nine women, every one slim and gorgeous, and all appearing to be under twenty-five. The show's promotion does mention that Cybill Shepherd – who is fifty-nine, and a mid-life boomer woman – is joining *The L Word*'s fourth season.[29]

While these representations are a long way from Lucille Ball and *The Lucy Show*, it has taken more than forty years to get this far.

Meanwhile, there are also hopeful signs in theatre. A traveling theatre project, featuring the work of six female playwrights, has been spearheaded by playwrights Donna Guthrie and Nancy Gail-Clayton. They invited American female playwrights who would be turning sixty in 2006 to submit one-act plays, with the proviso that they had to include complex roles for older female actresses

"We are such a youth-obsessed culture," says Guthrie. "So many times in plays the older woman is the cranky grandmother, eccentric aunt or the bitchy mother-in-law. When is the last time you saw a sexy or complex older woman role? I feel we have much to say."[30]

Yes, indeed. It is high time that TV writers and producers et al got on the same page as these playwriting women.

Greetings!

Sending funny cards on the occasion of birthdays and anniversaries is a common way of expressing affection and delight to close friends and family members. And even the ability to design one's own personal greetings cards on the computer doesn't seem to have made mailing greetings cards, especially birthday cards, any less important.

Upon closer examination, however, what we find in the cards available in the marketplace is an underlying acceptance of the cultural norm that says getting older is something to be avoided, denied, and mocked.

Although many people think that cards about older women are funny and harmless, upon serious examination we see more often than not, that they are anything but. Indeed, all too often they border on viciousness. I work in an office tower and recently went looking for a greeting card in the very ordinary card and gift shop at the mall level. The title of one card, in red on a yellow background, said, "OLD GIRLS gone WILD," and the sidebar picture depicted two older women in bathing suits above a caption reading "Sexy Senior Sweeties!" One of the women wears a bikini and her stomach and fleshy thighs protrude. Her breasts are large and sag down to her waistline, and there is a blackened bar across her nipples. To the right in large letters are the words, "Raw! Real! Revolting!" and at the bottom it says: "We deeply regret that this tape is UNCENSORED!" If the recipient has the stomach to look inside, the greeting she will read is: "You're not getting older, you're getting sexier. Happy Birthday."

Unhappy Birthday would be more appropriate for this card, which is so full of hatred for older women that it is grotesque. Yet another card shows three older women in front of a strip-teasing, muscular young male, and the caption indicates that two of the women have already had strokes while the third one is waiting her turn.

I did find one card that was quite funny, yet not insulting. It shows two older women, dressed in striped convict clothing, facing each other while pumping a handcart on a railway trestle. The caption is "Friends for Life."

The point that needs to be made is that depictions such as the first two I described are both ageist and misogynist. The same holds true for jokes: why are there so many mother-in-law jokes, but no father-in-law jokes? (There is even a spiked plant called "mother-in-law's tongue," but no "father-in-law's tongue".)

There is the joke about an older couple confined to separate beds in a nursing home, who hold hands for a moment before going to sleep each night. On one occasion, the woman does not offer her hand, and her spouse asks, "What's the matter?" She replies, "I've got a headache."

The "humor" here relies on the general acceptance of the false notion that older people are no longer sexual. More of this kind is to be found via e-mails entitled *FlowGo Fun Flush*, which arrive almost daily and unsolicited. If you click on the internet link they provide – which I once did – you will get "Grannies Gone Wild" and "Too sexy for My Granny" and another entitled "Geezer Pleaser." All are animated by hateful caricatures.

Political correctness enters here, and it is a slippery slope indeed. When Bill Maher, the American commentator, appeared on the CBC in June 2004, he made the point that "political correctness is sensitivity overblown to conceal truth."[31] What he was suggesting is that we should not throw the baby out with the bath water. For example, many people who have borne the brunt of racial prejudice use jokes as a way to relieve their discomfort. One joke about First Nations people concerns an Aboriginal man greeting Samuel de Champlain as he comes ashore on his first voyage up the St. Lawrence River. After they have a brief chat, the aboriginal man calls into the forest: "Come on out, we've been discovered!" A Scottish joke tells of an older woman who calls her local newspaper to insert an obituary. Asked what she wants to say, she replies, "Died, John McDonald, born June 1935, died September 2001." The clerk tells her that this is only one line and she will be charged for three lines, which is the newspaper's minimum. A pause ensues, then she says, "For sale, Morris Minor, 1983, 120,000 km, good condition, $2,000." Such in-group humor exists in most ethnic groups. It acknowledges certain traits and, by allowing people to laugh at their own trials and tribulations, eases tensions and strengthens bonds. In effect, it enhances group solidarity.

The problem arises when such in-group humor is picked up by those outside the group who, more often than not, utilize it to reinforce negative stereotypes. Consider this e-mail sent from one older woman to another. Referring to the long-term implications of modern drugs and surgical procedures, the sender writes: "Over the past few years more money has been spent on breast implants, penis implants, and Viagra than on Alzheimer's. In a few years we will have a lot of people running around with huge breasts and long dicks who won't remember what to do with them." This is hilarious within the context of a discussion taking place between two older women or men. But when younger people bandy this about, it serves to reinforce the widespread and false belief that all older people lose their memories.

We don't want to overdo political correctness, as this would make for a dull life. We can't and don't want to imagine a world without humor or the ability to laugh about and at ourselves, but humor or the ability to poke fun at ourselves can be a double-edged sword. What is acceptable in certain contexts is not acceptable within others.

Now You See Her, Now You Don't

"Quick: name five male film stars over age 50 still making box-office hits. Easy, right? Think Pacino,

Nicholson, Hopkins, Connery and Redford. Now name five current female stars over 50. Stumped? You're not alone . . ."[32] Even though researcher Hope Green only wrote this poser in 2001, in the five short years since then it has actually become easier to name five older female actors: a heartening example of how quickly things may improve given favourable circumstances and activism by media watch organizations. See if you can name five females movie stars over fifty – perhaps starting with Olympia Dukakis.

Because films play such an important role in popular culture, they can function as a weathervane to determine the cultural climate. As critic Dean Keith Simonton notes, "Presumably mainstream motion pictures largely reflect prevailing cultural attitudes about gender roles, norms, attitudes and expectations . . . Yet it must be admitted that films are not merely mirroring sociocultural images; *films also create them*" (emphasis added).[33] When one thinks of how much of the world, apart from North America – and especially Canada, of course – watches major US box office successes, it gives us some idea of how powerful and influential films can be.

The Lady Vanishes is both the title of a classic British film and the evocative subtitle of a study by Elizabeth Markson and Carol Taylor on older women in films. With this double entendre they suggest that films, a hugely popular form of mass media, tend to lack balance with regard to portrayals of and by older women. They examined films within the context of changing demography, increased life expectancy, and gender roles, their aim being to see if the portrayals of older people in US feature films had altered between 1929 and 1995 – a period of sixty-three years.

Using "the film mirror of aging" as a metaphor, they suggest that the mask of male aging differs sharply from that of female aging. Male movie masks deny physical aging, while female masks frequently exaggerate it. Markson and Taylor found that men were more likely than were women to be depicted as vigorous, employed, and involved in same-gender friendships and adventure, whether they were portrayed as heroes or villains.

Women were more often portrayed as rich old women, as wives, mothers, or lonely spinsters, and they were rarely central to the action. They concluded that "film roles have remained remarkably static in age and gender stereotyping."[34]

These critics also found that males and females age differently in films, that older men, Jack Nicholson for example, remains vigorous and achieving, while women tend to be of interest only if they are youthful. Patricia Mellencamp, another film critic, coined the term "chronological disavowal," meaning that women can be forty or fifty but they must look thirty. She refers to this as "double-whammy logic."[35]

This view is echoed by Sharon Waxman, who talks about the industry's obsession with youth and beauty, and indicates that there hasn't been much change. "The unforgiving nature of the close up . . . makes it even harder for women to sustain marquee status for any length of time . . . Even top actresses can't expect their turn in the spotlight to last much longer than a laser peel."[36]

Films are clearly kinder to older men, depicting them as still vigorous. In *Space Cowboy*, James Garner, Tommy Lee Jones, and Clint Eastwood are astronauts who come to the rescue of a failing flight mission, their youthful skills still operative. In *Grumpy Old Men*, Jack Lemmon and Walter Matthau depict older buddies who are still sexually active and both attracted to, of course, a beautiful younger woman. And anyone who watched the 1991 Academy Awards was treated to the spectacle of an aging Jack Palance doing one-armed pushups on the podium, while remarking that he could do this even without a woman under him. His real life desire to appear youthful is reminiscent of Gloria Swanson's movie portrayal of Norma Desmond, a fading older woman film star in *Sunset Boulevard*, who is desperate to stay young.

An interesting twist, and one referring to current male stars, such as Bruce Willis, fifty-two, Harrison Ford, sixty-five, and Sylvester Stallone, sixty-one, is provided by the *New York Times* of February 3, 2008 titled "Forever Hunky: Ageless Action Figures." The article points out that with today's culture of Botox, steroids, plastic surgery stars can appear ageless. Stallone, who they suggest may have discovered human growth hormones, can play the same role he did in 1982 and even look younger. Their take on it is that the viewing public wants these actors to stay young forever, and won't allow them to age.

In an amusing vein, an observer found that, in the early era of Hollywood glamour women "[they] were, in the politically incorrect lingo of times past, tough broads: Bette Davis, Joan Crawford, Rosalind Russell: "women with a career, an attitude and meaningful shoulder pads."[37]

Older women Oscar winners are scattered over the years: Jane Darwell as Ma Joad in *The Grapes of Wrath* in 1940, Lila Kedrova as a dying old prostitute in *Zorba the Greek* in 1964, and Geraldine Page in the *Trip to Bountiful* in 1985. Hardly a tsunami.

Another writer, discussing Markson and Taylor's more recent research in which they look at strong female portrayals from the 1930s to the present, compares how British and American older actresses have fared in the film industry. They feel that Hollywood seems to have an ongoing love affair with older British women, while it considers American actresses over the hill after forty. "British actresses seem to come out of the woodwork . . . I mean whoever heard of Judy Dench before the 1990s?"[38] Dench received an Oscar in 1998 at age sixty-three. However, the writers still suggest that in both Britain and Hollywood, older women tend to be shown in a negative light.

Happily, Helen Mirren won in the 2007 Oscar for Best Performance by an Actress in a Leading Role for her portrayal of Queen Elizabeth the Second. Also nominated were Judy Dench, age seventy-two, and Meryl Streep, fifty-seven; Mirren was sixty-one. Perhaps a watershed year for older women Oscar recipients and nominees is in the making.

Some movies can definitely be considered in the "backlash genre." Two earlier ones are clearly resentful of the women's movement. In *Fatal Attraction,* Glenn Close portrays an independent, sexually aggressive woman who trolls for men in bars. She finds one – married, of course, because she is a home breaker – and they begin a torrid affair. When he seeks to end it, she becomes totally unhinged and ends up being a danger to both him and his family.

It is not hard to read this as indicating that uppity boomer women seeking independence will only end badly, in this case by going stark, raving mad. They will also constitute a threat to the traditional family – and this film was made well before the current US traditional family credo of "Focus on the Family."

Another film in this backlash genre against feminism is *Baby Boom* starring Diane Keaton, who portrays a successful corporate woman who somehow gets landed with a baby. Of course, this leads her to find the true meaning of a woman's life – being a mother. She ends up finding herself in a home-based business making applesauce and happily minding the baby. The message? Biology is destiny.

Dealing with the more current versions of the backlash, Johanna Schneller, a Canadian movie columnist in a review titled "Shrieking Shrews? Give me a break," takes to task films that she feels are aimed at kicking powerful, successful boomer women in the head, so to speak.[39] Here is what she writes:

> "Helen Mirren, 60, Bitch Boss to Kate Hudson in *Raising Helen* (success = coldness), Holly Hunter, 48, Bitch Boss to Brittany Murphy in *Little Black Book* (success = back-stabbing). Sally Field, 59, semi-bitch boss to Reese Witherspoon in *Legally Blonde 2* (success = ambivalence). Let's not forget Sharon Stone, 48, Bitch Boss in *Catwoman* (success = insanity) . . . At first, the actress played by Glenn Close, 59, in *Heights*, looks like an exception . . . but her husband cheats on her, and she drinks too much (Success = misery)."

Of course, the definitive portrayal could be that of Meryl Streep as the Boss from Hell in *The Devil Wears Prada* (success = Satan), according to Schneller.

The Prada film, apart from Streep's terrific performance, has several penetrating moments, including how the dragon-lady, as she is referred to by her underlings, sets these younger women against one another. Her assistant, well-played by Anne Hathaway, makes a remark about her bitch boss to the effect that, if her boss was a man, she'd be thought of as only doing her job as a successful executive: a gendered double standard with which we are all quite familiar.

In another article, "A Culture Saturated with Sexism" (*Globe and Mail*, December 15, 2007), Schneller writes an astringent critique of a growing trend in films (and as she notes also in TV, the Internet, and Tabloids) to denigrate the female body, which in her opinion has reached ugly proportions.

Citing the film maker Josh Whedon, who said on his website "Women's inferiority – in fact, their malevolence – is as ingrained in American popular culture as it is anywhere" and further "I find it in movies, I hear it in the jokes of colleagues, I see it plastered on billboards . . . Women are weak, manipulative, somehow morally unfinished. The logical extension is that women are expendable . . . There is a staggering imbalance in the world that we all just take for granted."

These are heavy words, but it is exactly the "taking it for granted," meaning it is so totally ingrained in popular culture that we barely see it. This is a major boulder on boomer women's roadmaps – a boulder that needs cultural dynamite to shatter.

Is the Tide Turning?

With regard to gender attitudes and portrayals of midlife and older women in films, the winds of change have begun to blow: slowly, but they are blowing.

For example, *Thelma and Louise*, starring Susan Saradon and Geena Davis, a pivotal film about which much has been written, recognizes the importance of friendships between women. Thelma and Louise are "buddies." Unfortunately, their attempt to escape their male-controlled lives ends in their suicide – a pretty harsh resolution.

In *Fried Green Tomatoes*, two women – Jessica Tandy, who was eighty-two at the time, and Kathy Bates, who was forty-two, a boomer – play key roles. Markson notes that *Fried Green Tomatoes* "has often been described in the press as a 'female buddy picture' underscoring the lack of a woman's film comparable to the male 'buddy pictures'."[40] The film depicts the strong, positive influence of an older woman on a middle-aged woman.

The First Wives Club is about women getting even. Diane Keaton, Bette Midler, and Goldie Hawn are all mid-life boomers striking back at husbands who left them for younger women. While this is a feel-good film, a fantasy about the power of abandoned women to strike back, these women are all well-to-do matrons. The reality of most single, divorced women is far different than that of the women in this film.

More recently women actors, themselves baby boomers, have started to speak out. Jamie Lee Curtis displayed an air-brushed photo of herself, slim and trim, and then showed a photo of herself without airbrushing – love handles, thick thighs, and all. Her point was that this is what she and other mid-life women really look like. And at age forty-five, another well-known star, Andie Macdowell, said that she was saddened by Hollywood's obsession with youth, but that she has faith that, as baby boomers get older, they will demand to see women of their own age on the screen. She added, "I think it's changing a little bit, the baby boomers are now mature and they're gonna want something they can relate to – I hope."[41]

Without doubt, a prime example of positive change was the much touted film *Calendar Girls*, starring Helen Mirren, the older British actor at the leading edge of the boomer cohorts, who has had major roles in both film and television. *Calendar Girls* is an upbeat film about middle-aged women who come to feel that their bodies are perfectly suitable for nude photographs – in aid of a good cause, of course. It spoke to women, and few who saw it didn't relate immediately to the scene in which, on their way to being photographed, the women divested themselves of their bras so as not to be photographed with shoulder strap marks. There are now a number of other middle-aged and older women who are similarly posing nude for calendars, having been encouraged by this film not only to accept but to display their older bodies.

Laura M. Holson observed in the *New York Times* that Hollywood is a town ruled by conventional wisdom: "Teenage boys rule at the box office. The most marketable actresses are both pretty and young."[42] But she argues that filmmakers cannot continue to disregard "the demographic," referring both to roles for older women on the silver screen and the growing number of midlife boomer and older women buying tickets. Kate Winslet has summed it up succinctly: "It is very important to me that women on film are portrayed as real women . . . women that women in the audience can relate to and think 'I'm like that; that looks like me and all my friends'."[43]

Women are making some gains in another film category. Twenty-five percent of the acting nominees of both sexes for Oscars in 2004 had performed in films written or directed by women. And this is at a time when women represent only 7% of all Hollywood directors.[44] As another critic observed "aging is a culturally produced narrative of decline," and as I attempt to make clear, midlife and older women are certainly not declining.

Far from being ineffective, the social construction of aging as reflected in television and films is internalized by many women, starting when they are very young and continuing through their teens. In analyzing the culturally imposed fear of aging, Margaret Gullette comments, "If we dread old age as early as our thirties or forties, it is not because 'revulsion' is innate."[45] By this she means that revulsion is constructed: it is learned both overtly and covertly, obscuring women's heterogeneity, and great later life strengths. We are not born disliking aging women; we learn to do so.

The melding of ageism and sexism is extraordinarily destructive, and mid-life women need to recognize and resist these twin "isms" and not allow them to become self-fulfilling prophesies, so that they will be held back from fully developing their abilities in the twenty-five years or so that comprises the new stage of life ahead of them. This is vital for boomer women's roadmaps.

For the most part, older women of the present generation, my peers, accepted constant negative stereotyping and being told how to acceptably live their lives. They paid a high price for this, because so many of them lived restricted lives, as was made very clear in Betty Friedan's now classic book, *Feminine Mystique*.

A study entitled "Reinventing Aging" published by the Harvard School of Public Health, referring to the cultural construction of aging and boomer women's reaction to it, points out that "A key question . . . is whether boomers truly will break free of existing stereotypes, as many predict, or ultimately reinforce them."[46] While it is difficult to perceive that the more educated and more assertive boomer women will go along with the distortions of their lives as presented by popular culture, baby boom women and men do not constitute a homogenous entity: their cohort includes different social classes, religions, ethnicities, races, and sexual orientation, and these may be the deciding factors in how they approach the future.

When I was in the college system in the 1970s, a time when the women's movement was growing, I along with some like-minded women on faculty tried to change the language used in the courses being taught. Our goal was to eliminate the word "man," which functioned as an all-encompassing category that effectively excluded women. Curricula were strewn with courses bearing such titles as "Man and His World" or "The History of Man," and so on. Ours was a rather common sense request – or so we thought. But when at faculty meetings we suggested the need to change this, we were greeted with laughter and hoots of derision.

However, because of the persistence of feminists (who included some men), change did occur, and today it is usual to hear the phrases "he or she" and "hers and his" in radio broadcasts, TV, newspapers and everyday conversations. The point is it didn't take much more than a generation to accomplish this. And since we have already seen some resistance to ageist representations in films and television, surely there will be more connecting of the ageist dots in time, a niche on the roadmap which midlife boomer women could well occupy. I will give the last word to Julie Walters, the well-known British actor and one of the stars of *Calendar Girls* who said, "We're sort of the baby boomers, so there's a lot of us about. There's a big audience of us that aren't catered for . . . so women's stories are becoming slightly more common. Social change takes a long time, doesn't it? But I think that is changing."[47]

Things You Can Do As
A Boomer Woman Change Agent:

• Censorship begins at home. Train yourself to stop using words that demean yourself and other women, such as "old broads" or "hags."

• Don't refer to yourself or your peers as "old women," but rather as "older women." You'll be surprised at the difference this slight shift makes.

• When you see negative images of older women, try and do something about it. If, for example, it is a hateful greeting card, tell the store manager and suggest she/he stop offering them for sale and find more positive ones.

• If you wish to become more proactive about screen ads or images in magazines or newspapers or on TV that you find offensive, get in touch with whoever has the power to change it, no matter high up they are, to say it is unacceptable. Higher-ups (presidents, vice-presidents, directors) listen more carefully than mid or lower level employees. And be persistent. There are a number of media watch organizations you'll find on the net that are helpful.

• Support movies featuring positive images of mid-life women and those with mid-life actors and if possible, go with a friend and tell your group about it. Ticket sales count. Also, if you have an inner playwright waiting to emerge, write that TV script or play about mid-life women or older women you've always wanted to. You might start by thinking of your mother or grandmother(s).

References

1. Toni M. Calasanti and Kathleen F. Slevin, Eds. "Introduction" in *Age Matters: Realigning Feminist Thinking* (New York London, Routledge. Introduction, 2006), 3. See also Kevin E. McHugh "The 'Ageless Self': Emplacement of Identities in Sun Belt Retirement Communities," *The Journal of Aging Studies* 14, 1 (2000).

2. Margaret Cruikshank, *Learning to be Old: Gender, Culture and Aging* (Lantham: Rowman & Littlefield Publishers Inc, 2003).

3. Mary Grizzard, "Images of Aging Women" in *Handbook on Women and Aging*, ed. Jean M. Coyle (Westport, CT: Greenwood Press, 1997), 44.

4. Elizabeth W. Markson, "Sagacious, Sinful or Superfluous? The Social Construction of Older Women," in *Handbook on Women and Aging*, ed. Jean M. Coyle (Westport, CT: Greenwood Press, 1997), 53.

5. S. Jay Olshansky and Bruce Carnes, *The Quest for Immortality: Science at the Frontiers of Aging* (New York, London: W. W. Norton & Company, 2001), 28.

6. David Guttmann, "Reclaimed Powers Towards a New Psychology of Men and Women in Later Life," in *Later Life* (New York: Basic Books, 1987).

7. Elizabeth W. Markson, "Sagacious, Sinful or Superfluous? The Social Construction of Older Women" in *Handbook on Women and Aging*, ed. Jean M. Coyle (Westport, CT: Greenwood Press, 1997), 58.

8. Margaret Cruikshank, ibid., 140.

9. Matt Taibbi, "The Low Post: Hill on Fire," *Rolling Stone*, August 8, 2006, <http://www.rollingstone.com/politics/story/11111467/the_low_post_hillary_clinton_and_t...> (accessed November 3, 2007).

10. Jodi Enda, *The Mercury News*, January 20, 2008, <http://www.mercurynews.com/opinion/ci_8025804?nclick_check=1>

11. Jon F. Nussbaum et al., "Ageism and Ageist Language Across the Life Span: Intimate Relationships and Non-intimate Interactions," *Journal of Social Issues* 61, 2 (2005): 287.

12. Barbara MacDonald and Cynthia Rich, *Look Me in the Eye: Old Women, Aging and Ageism* (Denver, CO: Spinsters Ink Books, 1984), 11.

13. Frida Kerner Furman, *Facing the Mirror: Older Women and Beauty Shop Culture* (New York and London: Routledge, 1997), 94.

14. Ibid.

15. Erdman Palmore, "Sexism and Ageism," in *Handbook on Women and Aging*, ed. Jean M. Coyle (Westport, CT: Greenwood Press, 1997), 10.

16. Barbara MacDonald and Cynthia Rich, ibid., 77.

17. Harvard School of Public Health, *Reinventing Aging: Baby Boomers and Civic Engagement* (Harvard School of Public Health, Centre for Health Communication, Metlife Foundation, 2004), 5.

18. "Status of women weak on screen behind the scenes in the 1998-1999 Prime Time TV Season," *Media Report to Women* 27(1), Winter 1999: 15-17.

19. Tim Healey and Karen Ross, "Growing Old Invisibly: Older Viewers Talk Television," *Media, Culture and Society* 24 (2002): 105.

20. "More Television Dramas, and Growth of Cable TV, Redefine Women's Roles," *Media Report to Women,* Vol. 35, No. 1 Winter 2007, <http://www.mediareporttowomen.som/issues/351.htm> (accessed June 22, 2008).

21. Eva-Marie Kessler et al. "The portrayal of older people in prime time television series: The match with gerontological evidence." *Ageing and Society* 24, 4 (2004): 531-552. See also Tom Robinson et al. "Perceptions of negative stereotyping of older people in magazine advertisements: Comparing the perceptions of older adults and college students." *Ageing and Society,* 28, 2 (2008): 233-251.

22. *Globe and Mail,* July 14, 2002.

23. Harvard School of Public Health, *Reinventing Aging,* 138.

24. Scott D. Roberts and Nan Zhou, "The 50 and Older Characters in Advertising of Modern Maturity: Growing Older, Getting Better?" *Journal of Applied Gerontology* 16, 2 (1997): 209.

25. Janice Pearson, "Women's Health Matters – Aging, 2002," <http://www.Womensghealthmatters.ca/facts/quick_show_d.cfm?number=326> (accessed July 19, 2006).

26. Andrea Press and Terry Strathman, "Work, Family and Social Class in Television and the Construction of Post Feminism," *Women and Language* 16, 2 (1993).

27. Ibid.

28. Statistics Canada, *Women in Canada: A Gender Based Statistical Report* (5th Ed., Cat.no.89-503-XPE, 2006).

29. "Comments after Ellen" *The L Word*, 2006, <http"//www.afterellen.com?TV?thelword.html> (accessed September 9, 2006).

30. *Women's News*, September 28, 2006.

31. Bill Maher, appearance on the Canadian Broadcasting Corporation, June 10, 2004.

32. Hope Green, B.U.Bridge, "Film Study Shows Roles Favour Older Men, Stereotyped Women," Boston University, 2001, <http://www.bu.edu.bridge/archive/2001/10-05/filmstudy.htm> (accessed September 4, 2006).

33. Dean Keith Simonton, "The 'Best Actress' Paradox: Outstanding Feature Films Versus Exceptional Women's Performance," *Sex Roles* 50, 11/12 (2004): 781.

34. Elizabeth Markson and Carol A. Taylor, "The Mirror Has Two Faces: The Lady Vanishes," Aging and Society, 20 (2000): 137.

35. Patricia Mellencamp, "From Anxiety to Equanimity: Crises and general continuity on TV, at the Movies, in Life, in Death" in *Figuring Age: Women, Bodies and Generations*, ed. Kathleen Woodward (Bloomington and Indianapolis: Indiana University Press, 1999), 316.

36. Sharon Waxman, "Fade to Black: Women's Roles in the Movies," <http://www..discoverkate.com/Articles/ 20010303_iht-fadetoblack.html> (accessed June 5, 2005).

37. *Media Report to Women*, Winter 1993: 7.

38. Hope Green, op.cit.

39. Johanna Schneller, "The Movie Goer," *Globe and Mail*, June 2, 2006, R8.

40. Markson, "Sagacious, Sinful or Superfluous," 66.

41. Associated Press, *Vancouver Sun*, February 19, 2004.

42. Laura M. Holson, "Ideas and Trends: Aging Gracefully – And the Winner is . . . the Older Women," New York Times, January 18, 2004: 1-2.

43. "A Blast of Fresh Air," *Sunday Times*, October 29, 2006, <http://www.timesoutline.co.ul/article/0..2101-2424733.html> (accessed October 30, 2006). For a less encouraging view of directors and other women 'behind the scenes' in Hollywood, see "Film Directing is still a man's world" <http:www.latimes.com/entertainment/news/movies/la-et-goldstein202-2008may 20,0, 19432...> (accessed May 20, 2008).

44. Molly Haskell, "Has Film Come to Terms with Feminism?," *The Guardian*, March 5, 2004, <http://film.guardian.co.uk/story/0,12930,1162074, 00.html> (accessed May 6, 2005).

45. Margaret Morganroth Gullette, *Declining to Decline: Cultural Combat and the Politics of Midlife* (Charlottesville and London: University Press of Virginia, 1997), 94.

46. Harvard School of Public Health, *Reinventing Aging*, 132.

47. David German, "Older Women Grab Screen Times in New Films," <http://www.topnews.com/index/php?sid=152016&nid=114> (accessed June 5, 2005).

Chapter Two

The Peter Pan Principle:
Mega-Beauty Industries

It is not while beauty and youth are thine own
And thy cheeks unprofaned by a tear
That the fervor and faith of a soul can be known
To which time will but make thee more dear.

— *Believe Me if All Those Endearing Young Charms,*
Thomas Moore, Irish Melodies, (1808-1834)

The social construction of aging and its representation through popular culture is especially relevant for mid-life women who are under pressure from demeaning cultural practices and negative stereotypes. How midlife women deal with certain aspects of these pressures is evident in the ways they respond to constant urgings for them to assess their physical appearance and the measures – in some cases, drastic measures – which they take to present and maintain an aura of youthful beauty. Such measures are stumbling blocks on the roadmap to empowerment, and thus deserve not only attention but active resistance.

In their introduction to their appropriately titled book, *The Fountain of Youth*, editors Stephen Post and Robert Binstock tells us that anti-aging interventions to "slow, arrest and reverse phenomena associated with aging – have been part of human culture and societies since early civilizations."[1] Tracing these practices back to Babylonian times, they describe such bizarre operations as grafts from the testicles, ovaries, or glands of animals, cell injections from the tissues of newborn or fetal animals, and various elixirs. However, lest we begin to feel superior, the authors note that many practices continue in modern times and some new ones have been added. In fact, "the marketing and use of anti-aging products and services claiming to prevent, retard, or reverse aging have skyrocketed in recent years."[2] Noting the large role of the Internet in this trade, they go on to state that "increased consumer interest in [anti-aging efforts] appears to be fueled by their appeal to baby boomers trying to preserve their youthfulness as they approach old age as well as older persons attempting to rejuvenate themselves."[3] How accurate is this assessment, especially in relation to the focus on mid-life women as they age?

The Anti-Aging Pressure Cookers

"Every time I look in the mirror I see my mother" is a comment often made by midlife and older women. I have made it myself, though in my case it is my father I see in the mirror. The underlying text is discomfort because the reflection shows a somewhat older face, an unease that is not too surprising given the many ways in which women learn to fear advancing years.

But gender-linked age inequalities take on disproportionate emphases for longer living women, and are reflected in the oft-heard comment that men's "facial lines" represent character while women's "wrinkles" represent deterioration, loss of sexuality, and general uselessness.

Martha Holstein, in an insightful analysis of what she calls "the cultural devaluation of older women's bodies," amusingly admits her own response to this situation when, for example, she refuses an offer of a seat on a bus because she doesn't want to be placed in the categories of "old" or "less than." In "A Feminist Perspective on Anti-Aging Medicine" she writes, "Almost in defiance I pull out a book or an article to prove that I am still 'with it' (as if the person cares what I'm reading)."[4]

This is no doubt a common response on the part of women to the negativity of the cultures in which they are raised. Having an older visage and body within the current youth-defined environment means that a woman's worth within society is often appraised according to her appearance. A woman in her early sixties who was a member of one of my focus groups admitted "I know it is wrong, but I do try to look 'hip' as my daughter calls it – like by wearing skinny glasses and streaking my hair."

Women's self-appraisals have been conditioned by what is referred to as the "male gaze"; that is, she judges herself according to how she perceives herself to be judged by males and by other women who are similarly conditioned. In addition, older women see themselves through youthful eyes, and as a result, writes Holstein, "we are doubly objectified as we internalize both the male gaze and the gaze of youth."[5] A double whammy. If we think of diagrams of DNA, we can visualize this process as a sort of cultural double helix.

Women can internalize these both negative and contradictory impulses in myriad ways. One widely recognized technique is referred to as the "mask of aging," which was expressed by one of the focus group women as "I may be old on the outside but I'm young inside." Another woman in the group told me, "I may look old, but I don't feel old." This common psychological tactic splits one's outward appearance from one's inner subjectiveness: "they" are old, but "I" am not. In current TV talk-show jargon this would be referred to as being "in denial." The distancing of a woman's older self from others who are "really old" is paralleled by trying to achieve constant youthfulness through engaging in such anti-aging activities as cosmetic surgery and the pursuit of what is termed "the new agelessness." The writers Calasanti and Slevin, referred to in the previous chapter, writing on the edict to remain youthful note "In this sense successful aging means not aging, not being 'old' or at least not looking old" (anti aging medicine will be discussed further in the following chapter).[6]

In "The Seductiveness of Agelessness," Molly Andrews describes this mindset as "socially induced schizophrenia," that is, as trying to live up to a cultural ideal by splitting yourself psychologically between what you look like and what you think (and are told) you should look like. The woman caught up in this impasse can "neither stay the same as she has been, for physical aging is inevitable, nor, having internalized the value of an ageist culture, can she move forward and embrace her future as an old person."[7]

This distancing tactic can itself be seen as a form of ageism. I interviewed an older woman, herself a psychologist, who put it this way: "I think it is a kind of ageism to distance oneself from the 'others.' When walking down the street, I catch a glimpse of myself [in a store window], and for a fraction of a second I do not recognize this person. Yet I recognize the 'inside me all the time as being the same me as I always was with minor alterations due to maturity. I think perhaps at the root of that is our own sense of continuity of personality –'I'm still the same inside as I always was.'"[8]

This idea of the continuation of self is in line with the notion that, as we age, we are constantly developing. Of course, we change as we get older, but our core – what most of us think of as our values, what we believe in and the things that are important to us – remains basic, even though it may take a different shape and be expressed differently than it was in our youth or as we mature.

That was then, This is now

Hand in hand with advertisers, the beauty industries are well informed about this "split" between women's actual appearances and how they are pressured and pressure themselves to appear, and they capitalize on it in major ways. But the social standards of beauty and the markers by which women judge their appearance and evaluate to what degree that they are conforming to social expectations have changed historically and culturally. And Diane Myers, in her article "Miroir, Memoire, Mirage," observes that it helps to bear in mind that beauty is not an inborn property, and that ideals of beauty are culture-bound and historicized, her point being that standards change, including today's.[9]

Our perceptions of human beauty have undergone many modifications over the past 5000 years. In some tribal cultures, the symbols of beautification include tattoos and body scarring by both men and women as they seek to make themselves attractive to peers, ready themselves for marriage, and show appropriate religious/spiritual behavior and tribal allegiance.

Among some African tribes, widened noses are admired, so noses are broadened during childhood, then decorated. In both Africa and South America, lip plugs – wooden labrets several inches in length – have been used to enhance attractiveness and also render the wearer unappealing to slave traders, a pretty canny motive. Clearly, kissing as we know it was not practiced there! Body piercing has involved placing bone ornaments in noses and ear lobes as markers of attractiveness.

Some tribal societies prefer plump women while others prefer long pendulous breasts; still others prefer upright breasts. In Sudan, Nuba girls undergo painful scarring.[10]

Genital mutilation, which sadly is still performed, represents the ultimate barbarity committed in order to change a girl's body to conform to male cultural and sexual imperatives.

Hair beautification can include smearing dung and grease on the head and not washing it for weeks. (Can you imagine writing a TV shampoo ad for that one?)

In Mangbidu, women arrange braids over a cylindrical metal frame affixed with needles and bones.[11] In Burma and Thailand, women's necks are elongated, being stretched by half-inch-wide brass rings, with as many as ten of them used (perhaps the artist Modigliani, famous for his paintings of long-necked women, was inspired by them.) And we are all familiar with the horrors of Chinese foot binding, which thankfully is no longer tolerated. Interestingly, however, as I researched these early beauty practices and "googled" such key words as "tribal," "women," and "beauty," what also came up were many ads for tattooing and body piercing in the here and now, a fact of life that many boomer women are certainly acquainted with in their teen-aged offspring. *Plus ça change.*

In her groundbreaking study *The Beauty Myth*, Naomi Wolf asserts "the qualities that a given period calls beautiful in women are merely symbols of the female behavior that that period considers desirable: *The Beauty myth is always actually prescribing behavior and not appearance* (emphasis Wolf's)."[12] Following the industrial revolution and the development of public and private spheres, men's role involved going out and making money while women's role involved domesticity. As the middle class grew, Victorians began to view women as creatures of leisure. Wolf depicts women's work as repetitive and time-consuming, including "painstaking tasks such as needlepoint and lacemaking."[13] Though it sounds comical now, this activity probably allowed women to express some creativity. Older women may remember the 1949 movie *The Heiress*, with Olivia de Havilland grimly working away at her needlepoint while her betraying lover, Montgomery Clift, bangs on the door seeking entrance.

Suffragettes, rebelling against this trivialization of women's abilities and this repression of their intelligence and energy, fought for women's votes and were met with scathing denunciations. To set them apart, these Victorian feminists were frequently described as "big, masculine wom[en], wearing boots, smoking . . . cigar[s] and swearing like . . . trooper[s]."[14]

Meanwhile, what was culturally defined as feminine beauty was dramatically altering other women's natural appearance. The whalebone corset was an unnatural attempt to rearrange women's bodies into an idealized hourglass figure. Some enthusiasts went so far as to remove one of their ribs to better effect a wasp-waistline.[15] In Ruben's time (1577-1640) women were admired for being plump, while flappers in the 1920s strove for slim bodies and flat breasts. And during the Great Depression of the 1930s, most women were more concerned with putting food on the table than beautifying themselves.

But ideals of beauty change not only historically and cross-culturally, but intra-culturally as well. Scanning fashion magazines such as Vogue in the latter part of the twentieth century reveals an astonishing variety of images of idealized beauty.

However, what has not changed, and if anything has become more intense, are women's responses to current standards of beauty, and this is a fact of great significance to mid-lifers' roadmaps. It appears that in order to meet cultural expectations, women may be acting to please others more than to please themselves. As Wolf notes, "the beauty myth is not about women at all. It is about men's institutions and institutional power."[16] And since the mid-twentieth century, this institutional power has relied more and more on the ability of corporations to shape and commodify current standards of beauty, now aided by the proliferation of technology, including, of course, the internet. But it is not only baby boomer women, living as they do in a youth-worshipping environment, who are affected by the intertwining of corporate mass advertisinand the corporatization of mega-beauty industries. Increasingly, it is young girls – even toddlers – who are being habituated to the commodification of beauty.

Early to Bed, Early to Rise – Advertise, Advertise, Advertise

The title of this section is a play on a slogan by Ray Kroc, the founder of McDonalds, and a testimony to the now globalized restaurant empire, recognized worldwide by its golden arches branding.

It is not just the scope and sheer pervasiveness of advertising power that is frightening; it is also its increasing intensity.

And, to no one's surprise, corporate advertisers have recognized the tempting possibilities of the aging boomer women's market. In an article entitled *Marketing Focus: Targeting Boomer Women*, Alex Miller tells us "While the bulk of ad impressions aimed at women have traditionally skewed toward 18-34 year olds, advertisers are starting to come around to the notion that there's plenty to gain by appealing to mature women. After all, women ages 40 to 50 generally have more disposable income than younger counterparts."[17] Two Australian social researchers have pushed this a bit further by pointing out that marketers have to shift their focus from targeting Generation Y to those between 45 and 54, because boomers and seniors are increasing their share of discretionary spending.[18]

Mass advertising, now global in scope, means mass consumerism. Nielson Media research stated that in 2002, men watched television for four hours and twenty-two minutes per day, while women watched for four hours and 58 minutes per day.[19] It appears that time spent online is now catching up with time spent watching TV, according to a 2006 Jupiter Research report (the net, of course, includes advertising).

Writer Jean Kilbourne tells us in her book, *Deadly Persuasion: Why Women and Girls Must fight the Addictive Power of Advertising*, that "the average American is exposed to at least three thousand ads every day and will spend three years of his or her life watching television commercials. Advertising makes up about 70% of our newspapers and 40% of our mail."[20] These are startling statistics, and one tends, at first, to resist them; however, when we consider all possibilities for exposure, they come more sharply into focus.

How many times a day and in how many ways are we exposed to advertising? It is in your face and all over the place: television; radio; the Internet; newspapers; magazines; signs inside and outside cars, trucks, and buses; departure areas for buses, trains, and airlines; billboards; neon signs; the sides of buildings; inside malls and stores; on shopping carts; in elevators; junk mail and flyers; concert and other event programs; sports events, with advertising on the perimeters of the fields (think Olympics or baseball or football); around the boards or in the ice of hockey rinks; branded clothing on sports players; the labels on most of our articles of clothing; T-shirts and other garments that display logos; match boxes; movie rentals; rock videos; at films and in films themselves (in the trade, this is referred to as "product placement." An actor holds a coke, flips a cigarette out of a branded box or drives a particular make of car. There is even an award given for the best placed product.) And on and on it goes.

Actually, the common act of buying an article of clothing, such as a T-shirt, then wearing it and thereby advertising the name of the maker printed on the front of it approaches the surreal. The customer is establishing that she and this designer name brand are inseparable, and this is somehow thought to give the customer status. Never mind that most of these articles of clothing are all made the same way and likely in similar places, "outsourced" to some Third World location, after which a variety of brand-names are added to the exact same products.

Very recently another variation has been added to the customer-brand-name-symbiosis: getting tattooed with a brand-name logo – it appears even on the forehead – so that the person and the brand name are literally inseparable.

And it may not stop there. According to an article published in the *The Globe and Mail*, two Caltech researchers are investigating the effect of marketing – perhaps the most pervasive force in our consumer culture – on the most complex object in the world: the human brain. The article notes that what is being sought are ways to more effectively harness the neural circuits of reward and desire. They even have a name for this: it is called neuromarketing.[21] And to think we feared 1984 . . .

We tend to disassociate ourselves from the advertising phenomenon by asserting that we don't pay any attention to its influences; however, according to Jean Kilbourne, advertising works precisely because we don't think it works on us. One has only to look at its effects on boomer women who are aging and who are already living within a culture that is hostile to aging. Mass advertising has created a population willing to take up and imitate any number of "received images of femininity."[22] Ads play on women's fears of aging, their dissatisfaction with their own images and appearance (the received images).

They commodify almost every bodily feature separately: skin, hair, eyes (lashes, lids and brows), nose, mouth, lips, teeth, chin, neck and downward to the breasts, waistline, hips, buttocks, legs and feet, toes and nails. Perhaps the soles escape, probably because hardly anyone sees them. The message is that you, as a woman, have a need and/or a problem that our product(s) can fix. In this way, corporate advertisers who target women's insecurities establish a constantly renewable, never-ending cycle.

It works like this: first, the hucksters recognize that fears are already there, for example, *I'm too fat*. Second, they establish the consumer's vulnerability through the manipulation of said fear: The fatter you get, the less attractive you'll be. Third, they offer ways to fix "the problem": "We'll take care of this for you" or

"We have the solution to your problem, just take Magician's brand diet pill or energy drink." In this way, the industry, bent on creating ever new markets while re-jigging the standard targets already established as "new and improved" (Magicians's Plus) and continuing to invent yet more territories to conquer.

Never too Early to Learn

As Margaret Gullette states in "Older Women Unite! Gray is Gorgeous": "Our commerce in aging with its billions of dollars reminding us daily that we need expensive surgeries and pills . . . makes aging-past-youth a curse in America."[23] This is helped along by advertisers that are placing increasing emphasis on marketing to younger and younger targets and thus manipulating the buying habits of their parents, particularly their mothers.

Little girls learn very early that being called pretty or cute is a compliment that makes everybody – themselves, their parents, grandparents and friends – proud. They learn the importance of their appearance, their body and weight, all of which are measured against the going cultural standards of beauty.

In a recent book provocatively titled *Born to Buy*, Juliet Schor discusses how marketing and advertising have been influential in transforming children into autonomous and empowered consumers. Schor states,

"Today, marketers create direct connections to kids, in isolation from parents and at times against them. The new norm is that kids and marketers join forces to convince adults to spend money."[24] Furthermore, she suggests that children have replaced active pursuits with shopping and watching more television and now, as we have just seen, going online. One newspaper review of Schor's book is accompanied by a picture of two three-year-olds, a girl and a boy who are referred to as "tykes." The little girl is wearing a Gap sweater, and the boy, a bomber jacket. One could say that in this instance gender equality had been achieved.

Those of us still trying to figure out what a "training bra" does can now abandon that pursuit, given more recent developments. In the reportedly fourteen billion dollar spa industry in North America, luxury spas for kids and teens are an important and growing market. Here, children as young as six can choose from the "Spa Kids Menu" with options that include: a manicure (20 minutes) for $18 (US); polish (change only) for $10; Tutti-Frutti Manicure Delight (20 minutes) for $25; pedicure (forty minutes) for $40; teen make-up instruction (time varies) for $50. There is also skin exfoliation; this for nine-year-olds, mind you. And, thoughtfully, togetherness is recognized, because for $65, one can sign up for a parent and child massage.[25] And "summer fashion design camps" are available for girls who ache for haut couture, reportedly at ages seven to thirteen. One model, aged eleven, is described as wearing a "pink crushed-velvet jersey dress with pink tulle, iridescent sparkles, black lace and corset detailing."[26] At least the supermarkets that provide the familiar miniature shopping carts for children, decorating them with small flags that declare "customer in training," are being honest about their intentions.

Boys are now also a market niche. Apparently, "Mom just doesn't know what to do" when her son stops smelling like baby-powder, but Proctor & Gamble – among others – do know, and they are there to help. Calling their product line OT (short for overtime, a familiar sports phrase), they offer shampoo, hair gel, pomade, body wash, deodorant, and antiperspirant (two fragrances, one smelling a bit like musk, the other a cross between lime and honeydew melon). As one especially sensitive consultant noted, no boy wants to smell like strawberries or tutti-frutti.[27]

However, there is another and far more disturbing side to the frivolities just described: the increasing sexualization of children, especially girls. Kilbourne discusses what she calls the "pornification" of ads, citing Pepsi, Prada, and Calvin Klein among others.[28] Calvin Klein, whose highly sexualized ads border on pornography, had to pull them twice – once in 1995 and again in 1999 – which, of course, gave his company huge media coverage.

Pornography has crept stealthily into our cultural world, and we have become inured to, for example, women's (and to some degree men's) revealing underwear ads, with lingerie being increasingly risqué but increasingly less shocking. In the 1950s, women bared about 20% of their bodies in advertisements. Now it is close to 60%.

A prime example of the sexual exploitation of images of little girls is nowhere better exemplified than in the so-called "beauty pageants" for very little girls. They are dressed up as female adults, wearing heavy make-up and appearing in sexy outfits suitable for women many years older. They mince about, mimicking women's stylized runway walks and gestures, often singing popular adult tunes. These pageants can only be termed grotesque. Their chief attraction is the sexualization of these children and this is far from harmless. The tragedy of six-year-old JonBenet Ramsay is immediately evoked, a depressing tale that has been widely reported.

A comprehensive and disturbing study titled *Report of the APA Task Force on the Sexualization of Girls* (The American Psychological Association, 2007), leaves no doubt about the degree to which a hypersexualized American popular culture affects girls, some as young as four to eight years old (one of a myriad of examples cited are of lingerie manufacturers who are selling thongs for this age group). The report analyses: advertising, products for sale, the media, music videos, music lyrics, dolls, movies, cartoons and animation, magazines, sports media, video/computer games, and the internet. In their words, "Massive exposure to media among youth creates the potential for massive exposure to portrayals that sexualize women and girls and teach girls that women are sexual objects."[29] The effects of such massive exposure leads the researchers to state: "Finally, the sexualization of girls may also contribute to the trafficking and prostitution of girls by helping to create a market for sex with children."[30] It is difficult, in fact shocking, to recognize that a sexualized pop culture could be this pernicious.

Girls and teens who are concerned – or more often obsessed – with their appearance have been convinced of the importance of being thin, having very likely been teased and taunted if they were heavy, or what is culturally considered to be heavy. Reports are replete about young girls, some in fourth grade, who are dieting, and twelve - thirteen year olds trying to lose weight by vomiting, using laxatives or taking diet pills. One Canadian study of girls aged ten to fourteen found 29.3 percent of girls aged ten to fourteen were trying to lose weight.[31]

But this is no longer news. As Kilbourne says, "Anorexia . . . is a disease with a complicated etiology and media images probably don't play a major role. However, these images certainly contribute to the body-hatred so many young women feel and to some of the resulting eating problems, which range from bulimia to compulsive overeating."[32] A good case can be made that the anorexic-looking fashion models of the mid-1990s had a huge influence on teenaged girls. An article written by one female teenager says in part, "Teenagers are under a lot of pressure to succeed and fit in . . . They are led to believe that if they are thin they will be accepted. Since many teenagers are constantly buying teen or fashion magazines, the images of emaciated models appearing in those magazine only reinforce their belief that in order to be happy, successful and accepted, they must be thin." She goes on to say that if girls love who they are, then they will be less likely to try to attain society's unattainable "ideal" body image.[33]

Another observation on this subject is made by Mara Kates—young daughter of the *Globe and Mail*'s food critic Joanne Kates—who was diagnosed with anorexia at fifteen. She reflects that, "As far as I know, it is pretty much impossible to go through life without feeling bad about yourself at one point or another. And eating disorders are just one sad way to bolster our self-worth."[34]

In the 1970s, the measuring stick (no pun intended) used for models was 8% under normal body mass index (BMI); in 2002, it ranged between 14% and 20%.

In July 2006, a report on the first medical study of websites that promote anorexia as a lifestyle choice was published in the *Globe and Mail*. It called on Canadian healthcare professionals and parents to be alerted to the danger of such sites, and the language developed by them and their users – words like "thinspo," short for "thinspiration" – in addition to their waif-like images. They even promote songs with lyrics that include "As long as we're emaciated, tastes outdated, yeah, everything will be fine."[35] In addition to the dangers to health, there is also the issue that girls are denied seeing a range of ordinary body sizes and shapes in the images they view as they grow up.

Eating disorders were not prevalent when I and my peers were teenagers – when putting food on the table was the major concern – so it is difficult not to see a connection between eating disorders and the constant depiction of stick-thin women in media images.

A hopeful sign that things may be changing for the better occurred in September 2006 in Madrid, when a ban was placed on super-thin or "melba toast thin models" at a prestigious fashion show. Other fashion centres are being urged to follow suit. But if the thin worm is turning, it will have to do a full one-hundred-eighty-degree turn to effectively counteract the thin-is-in culture.

Marking Ourselves Down

In the 1986 movie *Ruthless People*, the wonderful comic actor Bette Midler portrays the kidnapped wife of a wealthy Los Angeles man. When her inept kidnappers ask for a large ransom and, failing to get it, ask for less, Midler is shocked. "I'm being marked down," she says. In much the same way, midlife boomer women are "marked down" and devalued within our ageist society. Of course, we all admire beautiful young people, their glowing skin, tight abs, unmarked faces and so on, but we don't stay young forever, although for many of us this is not for lack of trying.

But women also mark themselves down. They internalize their own negative assessments of their appearance and make fun of themselves with frequent self-deprecatory remarks. How many times have you heard a woman describe her legs as too thin or too thick? Or describe herself as a spindleshanks or thunder thighs or tell you she is bowlegged, knock kneed, flat-footed, or pigeon-toed, that she has bony feet, thick ankles, feet too wide or too narrow (can never get shoes to fit) or that her arches too high? Such expressions of perceived inadequacy and dissatisfaction have a multiplier effect when applied to the whole body. We are either too big or too small or too something. Even Marilyn Monroe, the sex-goddess of the 1960s, who was groomed to play the dangerous "blonde bombshell" and measured 36-24-36, said of herself: "Everyone's laughing at me. I hate it. Big breasts, big ass, big deal. Can't I be anything else?"[36] Fortunately for Monroe, she was full-figured when it was "in" to be that way. Today, with many women physically unable to reach the goals of the thin-is-in culture, fashion designers have adjusted sizes to accommodate the sought-after slender image. They call this process "vanity sizing," a name that pretty well says it all. What was a size fourteen some time ago is now a size twelve, a twelve is a ten, and so on. There is also a size zero – the purpose of which escapes me. Surely to be "size nothing" suggests that one is either invisible, or dead. But it doesn't stop there. Apparently a size sub-zero is on the horizon to accommodate anorexic young women.

The effectiveness of cultural images that affect almost all women was highlighted dramatically in a global study that was released on September 19, 2004. Entitled *The Real Truth about Beauty: A Global Report*, this study, sponsored by Dove Soap, found that only 1% of Canadian women and only 2% of women worldwide consider themselves beautiful. Nearly half (47%) of those surveyed described their weight as "too high," while in Canada that number climbed to 54%; 63% strongly agreed that women today are expected to be more attractive than their mothers' generations were, and 26% had considered plastic surgery. Calling this "shocking and heartbreaking," Professor Susie Orbach commented, "Women have an inability to feel like they count in the culture of beauty."[37] If this is representative of how women measure themselves on a beauty scale, it isn't too hard to imagine that adding aging to the mix is unlikely to produce more positive results.

The purpose of this study was to produce a more diverse portrayal of women in popular culture. Of course, given that it was sponsored by a manufacturer of beauty soap, some skepticism is in order, but Dove does seem to be following through. A second report, released in February 2007, *Beauty Comes of Age,* showed higher numbers of mainly boomer women (86%) were proud of their age, though 91% criticized the lack of images of beautiful women over fifty.

An Oprah show in February 2007 featured a half dozen women – most in their fifties, though a couple were in their early sixties – who had been photographed in the buff by Dove and were proud of their appearance. The not-good news is that during this Oprah show the photographed women submitted to a "makeover" with the audience seemingly in awe of how much younger they then looked.

I found this to be missing the point. Still, Dove's findings are an eye-opener if for no other reason than they make the point that our current standards of female beauty are so restrictive, that virtually 100% of women in the 2004 study felt they fall outside beauty's boundaries. However, the positive views of older women in the Dove reports are to be commended, and should be encouraging to mid-life roadmappers. Yet many of them continue to take the most drastic measures to achieve what is, of course, impossible: that is, staying the same.

The Cutting Edge

Discussing her own dread of reaching middle age in an ageist culture, the writer Vivian Sabchak offered this: "I'm prepared to die but not to look lousy for the next forty years."[38] I'm sure most women reading this will nod their heads in agreement, because there is no doubt that if one looks good, one feels good. But the lengths to which some will go to avoid evidence of aging and to achieve that elusive, perpetual youthful image have reached extraordinary proportions. There are two relatively major approaches to "not looking lousy for the next forty years," the first being the recent and growing field of anti-aging medicine, or age-management as it is called.

One proponent of this field is Dr. Alan Mintz, who said when interviewed on *60 Minutes*, "This is not about the fountain of youth . . . it's about staying in charge of my life and being productive."[39] While Mintz's anti-aging regimen includes exercise, good nutrition, vitamins and so on, it also has a highly controversial aspect: his patients inject themselves with steroids and hormones to maintain control of the aging process.

On the other hand, feminists and others interested in women's issues feel that the pursuit of agelessness or efforts to "reverse" it are based on the cultural imperative to not look old and on interventions based on the premise that aging is preventable.[40] Frida Furman asks, "If women must conform to external standards of appearance in order to meet cultural expectations, to what extent are they agents of their own decisions?"[41] In other words, if popular culture is itself ageist, and women internalize this "poisonous ageist propaganda," as one critic has called it, mid-life women in pursuit of agelessness set impossible goals for themselves. This view then is in opposition to Mintz's idea of being in control of one's aging.

Cosmetic surgery and other beautifying pursuits are now cashing in on women's (and increasingly men's) dread of appearing older, to the point where the cosmetic industry's global profit exceeds $30 billion.[42]

On a more individual scale, in recognition of the human desire to look good, and because looking good makes us feel good, it may be helpful, though simplistic, to think of anti-aging pursuits as a pyramid. Perhaps the base of the pyramid consists of things most women do to look good: using lipstick, eye makeup, makeup base and hair coloring, all of these being non-invasive. The next level would be taking injections such as botox and submitting to other non-surgical procedures. The apex of this pyramid is the more intrusive cosmetic surgery: going under the knife.

According to the American Society of Plastic Surgeons, 7.4 million North Americans had plastic surgery in the year 2000. This was a 198% increase over 1998, when statistics were first collected.[43] Baby boomer women are participating in large numbers: thirty-five to fifty-year-olds make up 44% of the patients, 33% of them being repeat customers. (Cosmetic surgery procedures can become addictive. Just think of Michael Jackson.) Men account for 14% of all cosmetic surgery procedures performed. One Canadian surgeon suggests that over 80% of his patients are women.[44] In Canada, there is little in the way of data, because private medical centres where most of the surgery is performed are not obliged to make reports.[45] However, the American Society for Aesthetic Plastic Surgery (ASAPS) reported a 444% increase in the total number of cosmetic procedures in the US between 1997 and 2005. They also reported that in 2005, Americans spent $12.4 billion for all procedures.[46] Since Canadian figures are generally 10% of US data, we can guess the figure for Canada to be around $1.2 billion. A more recent study, done at the University Campus of Los Angeles (UCLA) states: "According to the American Association of Plastic Surgeons nearly 11 million cosmetic surgery procedures were performed in 2006 – a 48% increase from 2000. Roughly 90% of cosmetic surgeries in 2004 were performed on women."[47]

In Canada, the top five cosmetic surgical procedures accounting for 67% of all cosmetic surgical procedures, are nose reshaping, liposuction, eyelid surgery, breast augmentation and facelifts. The top cosmetic non-surgical procedures, which account for 79% of all procedures, include chemical peel, sclerotherapy, microdermabrasion, botox injection, and laser hair removal. Examples of surgical fees include: liposuction, $2000 (Cdn); breast augmentation, $6000; breast lift, $6000; tummy tuck, $5000; and facelift, $8000.[48]

And now there appears to be a new wrinkle (pun intended) to add to the proliferation of anti-aging procedures and their influence on mid-life women. A Canadian survey conducted between May 2005 and April 2006 informs us that Canadians are still fighting the aging process and the battle with gravity, but now they are shifting their interest to non-surgical facelifts with 4285 procedures performed in 2004 (a 19% increase).[49] "Newer procedures such as the FeatherLift™ and ThreadLift™ as well as treatments involving electrical currents, injectable fillers such as Restylane® and Perlane®, non-surgical lifts utilizing Botox® and most recently, Restyland SubQ™ have penetrated the market. The demand is staggering, with a 325% increase . . ." The study suggests that non-surgical procedures are becoming the norm. It also reports that the typical patient is a female between the ages of thirty-five and fifty, and that women account for 83.5% of the market, with men making up 16.5% for both surgical and non-surgical procedures.[50] If this type of "youthifying" surgery continues, we won't know what getting older looks like. We'll have a bunch of people running around with thirty-year-old faces attached to eighty- or ninety-year-old bodies!

Whether or not one agrees with the points being made about mid-life boomer women's preoccupation with staying and looking young forever, the following certainly drives the point home. In a discussion of the remake of the film *Stepford Wives*, an article in the *New York Times* refers to the Stepfordian obsession with cosmetic surgery: "The knife begins these days with the first wrinkle. Along with collagen implants and Botox, summer beauty treatments now include toe-shortening and even pinkie toe removal – the better to fit into pointy shoes."[51] This cosmetic foot surgery, elsewhere referred to as "toe tucks" takes us back to the Victorian example (above) of the removal of a rib to achieve a wasp waistline.

Ads for cosmetic procedures are now commonplace. An advertisement in one Canadian newspaper showed a young woman's perplexed face with the following printed across it: "What are you more afraid of, needles or wrinkles?" This certainly plays on women's fears of aging. And now that makeovers are done live on television, the push for cosmetic procedures has been further reinforced. There are ads promoting cosmetic surgery in teen girls magazines, and I have been told by my teen granddaughter that some girls turning sixteen are asking for bust enhancement surgery as a birthday gift, an apparently not uncommon request.

But it is important to remember that all surgery involves some risk. In Canada, Olivia Goldsmith, a writer who once told an interviewer that her sole goal in life was "to change the culture so that older women are perceived as full beings,"[52] died from complications following cosmetic surgery. What irony. Fortunately, such consequences are rare. The American Society for Aesthetic Plastic Surgery urges those considering cosmetic surgery to make certain that they select an ASAPS surgeon who is certified by the American Board of Plastic Surgery. In Canada, people are urged to make sure that the Royal College of Physicians and Surgeons of Canada can certify that their surgeon has practiced plastic surgery for at least three years following board certification, and that she/he qualifies for hospital privileges.[53]

It should be made clear that there are sometimes compelling reasons for cosmetic surgery, and that it can bring important benefits, thanks to modern medical technology and to the skill and devotion of the surgeons who practice it. It is obvious that people born with a disfigurement, those who have suffered an accident, or those who have real or even perceived physical defects that adversely affect their lives can benefit enormously from such procedures.

At a less dramatic level, one midlife woman who had developed a deep furrow between her brows told me that she had injections to smooth it out. She feels this has made her face look much more relaxed, and she is delighted. Her feelings can't be disputed.

What is puzzling is the dogged pursuit of the unachievable goal of agelessness. The Canadian actor Catherine O'Hara indulged in a satirical send up called *For Your Consideration* when she played "fading B-list actress Marilyn Hack, a socially awkward and insecure performer so titillated by the thought she might be an Oscar contender for her latest role that she Botoxes herself almost beyond recognition when it comes time to promote the film." The review on All New Radio continued: "When a sausage-lipped, cap-toothed, frozen-faced and bleached-out O'Hara saunters onto a Leno-ish late-night talk show spilling out of a skin-tight mini-dress, the audience . . . broke into its loudest laughs."

O'Hara herself said, "But it is scary . . . You see these thirty-year-old actresses in Hollywood, very pretty women and they get work done and they end up looking like well-preserved seventy-five-year-olds."[54] We've all seen such women with frozen, stretched faces, barely able to smile or frown – a dreadful price to pay for seeking agelessness.

I talked to several mid-life boomer women about these procedures. One in her late forties was opposed to all cosmetic surgery or other such interventions. She found it "depressing that women do these sorts of things, letting themselves get sucked in by all the emphasis on looking young and can't accept that we all get older." Two other midlife women I talked to had surgery, and felt differently. One, who is fifty-nine, had a saggy or "turkey" neck, making her unhappy. Two years ago she had a "necklift" and also had her eyelids done at a cost of $10,000. She is glad she did it, feels she looks rested and would do it again. Curiously, she is against Botox and implants as they introduce foreign substances into the body. The other boomer woman that I talked to, also midlife, had a facelift. She says she now feels good about herself and is told she looks fantastic; she also happily reported that "men are now hitting on me."

I believe, although I do so reluctantly, that there is another compelling reason why midlife women seek facelifts or other "youthifying" procedures. Living in the here and now and given the enormous pressure on women to appear youthful at all times and at all costs, the question of choice becomes central.

What are the choices? Referring to the loss that getting older entails, Sandra Bartky points out in

"Unplanned Obsolescence: Some Reflections on Aging" that "the fact that these losses are in some ways 'socially constructed' does not mean that they are easily overcome."[55] Being born into a sexist and ageist society, a mid-life woman who is concerned with having and keeping a job, especially in a downsizing environment (never mind the prejudice of some employers against hiring older women employees), trying to look younger by having a facelift could be considered a career move. It is certainly an extreme measure, but perhaps an appropriate response to the manifold pressures to appear youthful. It is common knowledge that women color their hair for similar reasons. Fortunately, the development of non-surgical facelifts, noted above, presents a less drastic alternative.

These are all huge issues that aging midlife women face as they proceed with their roadmaps. The conundrums are labrynthian and full of contradictions. One goes round, as it were, in cosmetic circles trying to determine choices to deal with the lessons of popular culture which insist that looking older is a no-no for middle-aged women – and now increasingly for men. Not for a moment can anyone stand in judgment of people resorting to anti-aging methods, whether for professional or personal reasons.

The challenge for baby boom midlife and older women is to find a middle ground between a denial of aging and the negativity of an ageist culture that coerces them to keep looking young. And the paramount dilemma is that anti-aging measures are ultimately self-defeating. Given these constraints and then saying that women should recognize their inner values, accomplishments, and successes – while absolutely true – sounds like a stream of platitudes. However, the recognition of self-worth is the key not only for women growing older but for any successful endeavour. To be good at anything one undertakes requires self-confidence. It is true for teen-aged women incessantly pressured to look thin and reverting to harmful dieting methods. It is increasingly true for boomer parents and grandparents who are exposed to an advertising culture that has now moved down the ageline to toddlers. I think that young Mara Kates, referring to the influences on teenagers, said it as well as it can be said when she wrote "As far as I know, it is pretty much impossible to go through life without feeling bad about yourself at one point or another." What an indictment!

The very young are encouraged to look and act older, and midlife women are urged to look younger and younger. One wonders if there is ever a time to feel good about oneself. Given that these major contradictions are part of our daily living, it is small wonder that feelings of self-worth are hard to attain.

However, helpful suggestions may come from unexpected sources. One analyst of the Dove Soap-sponsored study remarked: "Once you get people out of that narrow box where they have to have these stunning visuals, the word beauty opens up to a broader meaning. Who you look at as beautiful can then be determined by the totality of the person – their character, their personality, their intelligence and their vivacity."[56]

Assertive boomer women are very different than their accepting mothers, and because they are now in the majority, they could make a big difference.

Even a giant advertiser, McDonald's, was vulnerable when boomers and others who follow good nutritional habits simply stopped patronizing them. It didn't take long before salads and less fat-saturated food appeared on their menus. Voting with one's feet is empowering and an important and realizable roadmap strategy. Mass advertising can beget a mass response. Midlife baby boom women are well-positioned to resist the carpet-bombing of negative advertising and similar cultural forces. While size matters, so does gender, and there are more than four million women boomers in Canada. They are in a prime position to change the male/youth gaze to an older women's/ beauty gaze. It is time to shift from an anti-aging environment to a pro-aging one. We can then, as Molly Andrews reminds us, move forward and embrace our futures as older women.[57]

Things You Can Do As
A Boomer Woman Change Agent:

- Make a lot of noise. If you see fashions in magazines that feature young, skinny women, harangue the manufacturers and urge them to recognize the growing mid-life women's market. Point to the 2007 Dove report as a model. Be positive in telling those who do feature mid-lifers realistically that you appreciate it. For example, the shopping channel in Canada regularly uses older average and larger-sized women as models.

- If you have decided to have cosmetic surgery or other cosmetic interventions, check the surgeon's qualifications carefully. Don't go to someone in a strip mall or a spa. The same thing holds if you decide to undergo procedures in another country, which a number of women now do.

- Many boomer parents have to deal with the difficulty of their teenagers being relentlessly exposed to "thin-is-in" images. Help young teenage women to "love themselves." Building their self-esteem and avoiding being hyper-critical will enhance their feelings of self-worth and bolster their resistance.

- Some magazines intended for teen-aged girls now advertise cosmetic surgery for them. If you object, in addition to getting in touch with the editors and telling them so, consider a blog on the internet to other parents similarly concerned.

- Don't mark yourself down by making derogatory references to your appearance. You are a role model to your kids, other family members, and co-workers, as well as your peers. Feel good about yourself and it will show.

- When you look in the mirror, instead of seeing your mother, see yourself. See your accomplishments, how much knowledge you've acquired, what a range of skills you have, how many people depend on you, how good you are for your family, for your friends, at your job or volunteer activity. You'll be surprised at how it all adds up.

References

1. Stephen G. Post and Robert H. Binstock, eds. Introduction to *The Fountain of Youth*, (New York: Oxford University Press, 2004).

2. Ibid.

3. Ibid.

4. Martha B. Holstein, "A Feminist Perspective on Anti-Aging Medicine," *Generations 25* (2001-02): 38.

5. Ibid., 40.

6. Toni M.Calasanti and Kathleen F.Slevin, Eds. "Introduction," *Age Matters: Realigning Feminist Thinking* (New York London,Routledge. Introduction, 2006), 3.

7. Molly Andrews, "The Seductiveness of Agelessness," *Aging and Society 19* (1999): 308.

8. Olive Johnson, personal communication, September 2004.

9. Diane Tietgens Myers. ed. "Miroir, Memoire, Mirage: Appearance, Aging and Women," *Women, Aging and Ethics*, (Urban: Lanaham, Rowman and Littlefield Publishers, 1999), 35.

10. Julian Robinson, *Quest for Human Beauty* (New York: W. W. Norton, 1998).

11. Nan McNab, *Body Bizarre, Body Beautiful* (New York: Fireside, 1999).

12. Naomi Wolf, *The Beauty Myth: How Images of Beauty Are Used against Women* (New York: Doubleday, 1991), 13-14.

13. Ibid., 15.

14. Ibid., 18.

15. Abu-Laden, Sharon McIrvin and Susan A. McDaniel, "Beauty, Status, and Aging," *Feminist Issues: Race, Class and Sexuality*, 4ed., ed. Nancy Mandell (Toronto: Pearson Education Centre, 2004), 118.

16. Wolf, *The Beauty Myth*, 13.

17. Alex Miller, "Marketing Focus: Targeting Boomer Women," March 2005, <http://publications.mediapost.com/index.cfm?fuseaction=Articles.ShowArticle & Art_aid+276...> (accessed September 7, 2006).

18. Simon Canning and Lara Sinclair, "End of the love-in," *The Australian News*, October 20, 2006, <http://www.Theaustralian.news.com.au/story/0,2087

6,20611300-28737,00.html> (accessed October 20, 2006).

19. <http://answers.google.com/answers./threadview? id=39247> (accessed October 8, 2003); Time Spent Watching TV (US) <http://answers.google.com.answers. threadview?id=392457> (accessed October 8, 2004).

20. Jean Kilbourne, *Deadly Persuasion: Why Women and Girls Must Fight the Addictive Power of Advertising* (New York: The Free Press, 1999), 58-9.

21. Jill Mahoney, "The Brave New World of Neuromarketing," *Globe and Mail*, September 10, 2005, A10.

22. Frida Kerner Furman, *Facing the Mirror: Older Women and Beauty Shop Culture* (New York and London: Routledge, 1997), 45.

23. Margaret Morgenroth Gullette, "Older Women Unite! Gray is Gorgeous," Women's E-News Commentary, November 10, 2004 <http://www.womensenews.org/ article.cfm/dyn/aid/2062/> (accessed November 14, 2004). See also <http://www.globalaging.org/ elderrights/us/2004/jokes.htm>.

24. Juliet B. Schor, *Born to Buy: The Commercialized Child and the New Consumer Culture* (New York: Scribner, 2004). See also Christopher Dreher, "Are Hip Tots Heading for Trouble?" *Globe and Mail*, September 25, 2004. p. 16

25. Doug Warren, "Pampered and Ticklish," *National Post*, February 21, 2004, PT6.

26. Gabrielle Giroday, "Fashion Design Camp Inspires the Tween Set," *Globe and Mail*, August 14, 2004.

27. Claudia Deutsch, "In the Armpit of a Boy," *National Post*, March 6, 2004, SP8.

28. Kilbourne, *Deadly Persuasion*, 281.

29. *Reference Report of the APA Task Force on the Sexualization of Girls, Washington, DC.* American Psychological Association, 750 first Street NE: 5. Available online at <www.apa.org/pi/wpo/sexualization.html>, 2007.

30. Op.cit., 34.

31. Gail McVey, et al. "Dieting among preadolescent and young adolescent females." Analyzes a study by the Canadian Medical Association Journal (CMAJ). May, 2004. http://www.cmaj.ca/cgi/content/full/170/10/1559. (Accessed 2/6/2007).

32. Ibid., 135.

33. Colleen Thompson, "Teenagers and Eating Disorders," <http://www.mirrormirror.org/teens.htm> (accessed May 18, 2004).

34. Mara Kates, "Words of Advice from Someone Who Has Been There," *Globe and Mail*, July 10, 2004, F8.

35. Alexandra Shimo, "Forums Promoting Anorexia Post Health Risk, Study Warns," *Globe and Mail*, July 8, 2006, A9.

36. Stephanie Smith, "Bombshell," *Body Politic and the Fictional Double*. ed. Debra King Walker (Bloomington: Indiana University Press, 2000), 160.

37. Misty Harris, "99 Percent of Canadian Women Wouldn't Call Themselves Beautiful," *Vancouver Sun*, September 29, 2004, A3.

38. Vivian Sabchak, "Scary Women: Cinema, Surgery, and Special Effects," *Figuring Age:Women, Bodies, Generations*, ed. Kathleen Woodward (Bloomington and Indianapolis: Indiana University Press, 1999), 200.

39. "Aging in the 21st Century," *CBS News*. <http://www.cbsnews.com/stories/2006/04/19/

60minutes/main1512855.shtml> (accessed September 25, 2006).

40. Holstein, op.cit.p. 40.

41. Furman, *Facing the Mirror*, 62.

42. "Industry Leaders, Analysts Forecast Cosmetic Plastic Surgery," <http://news.yahoo.coms?usnw/20060921? pl_usnw/industry_leaders_analyst_forecast_co...> (accessed September 28, 2006).

43. "Beauty by Design," *Overview: Cosmetic Surgery in Canada*, <http://www.cbc.ca/programs/sites/features/hm_cps,e tocsirgeru/overview.html> (accessed August 30, 2004).

44. Ibid.

45. Jane Armstrong, "TV Drives Plastic Surgery Craze," *Globe and Mail*. April 16, 2004, A11. See also on same page, Andre Picard, "Patients Should Know the Dangers of Going under the Knife."

46. "Survey Shows Canadians Choosing Non-surgical Options in Cosmetic Enhancements," <http:www.newswire.ca/ en/releases/archive/July 2006/13/c9261.html> (Cosmetic Surgury: National Data Bank, Statistics, The American Society for Aesthetic Plastic Surgery,

Expanded data for 2005). The Authoritative Source for Current US Statistics on Cosmetic Surgery.

47. "Huge Numbers Want Cosmetic Surgery, Study Finds," *Science Daily*, <http://www.ssciencedaily.com/releases/2007/1026162139.htm> (accessed October 28, 2007).

48. Ibid., 2.

49 Survey shows, op.cit. p.1

50. "The Medicard Report (2006) Survey Shows Canadians choosing non-surgical options in cosmetic enhancement," <http://www.neewswire.ca/en/releases/archive/July20 06/13c9261.html> (accessed September 29, 2006). This report comes from a medical finance company who report that 180 000 Canadians applied to them for financing. Their data is based on 2500 surveys sent out to board certified surgeons and physicians, as well as dermatologists and cosmetic surgeons and physicians throughout Canada.

51. <http://www,nytimes..com/2004/06/09/opinion/0990REN,htm>1?th> (accessed August 30, 2004).

52. Susan Schwartz, "The Sad, Ironic Death of Olivia Goldsmith," *Vancouver Sun*, February 4, 2004.

53. <http://www.google.ca/search?q=cache:z837cWCJ
IAYJ:Surgery.org/download/consumerbr..> (accessed
August 30, 2004).

54. All News Radio, <http://www.news1130.com/news/
entertainment/article/jsp?content=e091121A> (accessed
September 11, 2006).

55. Sandra Lee Bartky, "Unplanned Obsolescence: Some
Reflections on Aging," *Mother Time:Women, Aging and Ethics*,
ed. Margaret Urban Walker (Lanham: Rowan and
Littlefield Publishers, 1999), 69.

56. Harris, op.cit.

57. Andrews, op.cit.

Chapter Three

Where's the Rest of My Eyebrow?: Changing Health and Healthy Change

First, do no harm.
— Medical Maxim

If a midlife or older woman who goes to see a health practitioner is told that her uterus is attached to her brain, she will likely look around nervously for a quick escape route. But believe it or not, such was the wisdom existing not that long ago. Read on.

As we age, decline is inevitable and inevitably on the roadmap. In their book *Look Me in the Eye: Old Women and Ageism*, writers Barbara Macdonald and Cynthia Rich describe how they see older bodies: "Standing before the mirror in the morning . . . I see that the skin hangs beneath my jaw, beneath my arms . . . Below my stomach a new horizontal crease is forming over which the skin will hang like the hem of a skirt turned under . . . a hem not to be let down as when I was a child."[1] Aching joints, sagging breasts, lessening of vision and hearing, slower memory, liver spots, extra chins, loosening skin and other victories of gravity, along with shoving oneself up off the bed in the morning and climbing stairs more slowly are among the ways we experience aging bodies. Of all the changes to our anatomies, it seems that one in particular has a sense of humor: hair. It disappears, rearranges itself, or crops up unwanted where it did not exist before. For women, hair can thin and disappear from underarms and legs. The eyebrow comment in this chapter's title was made by a sixty-year-old woman who woke up one morning with part of an eyebrow missing. For older men, baldness is central to their aging concerns as they watch their hair recede or regroup. Of course, younger men also experience balding, but it doesn't have the same connotations. David Letterman, the TV talk show host, once remarked that the oblong shape left by his receding hairline reminded him of a bathmat. And there is the story of stripper Gypsy Rose Lee, who was performing well on in her career, when someone called out, "Have you still got it, Gypsy?" to which she replied, "I still got it, honey, only it's two inches lower" – a good-natured remark about acceptance of her changing body.

The point is that yes, we all experience decline, but it happens differently to different people at different rates and in different ways. We have all known women in their sixties who have more health difficulties than do women in their eighties. My own mother, all five feet of her, decided at age ninety-one to rearrange her very heavy wrought iron dining room furniture by herself, and did so successfully.

For midlife women, an aging body can be a source of anxiety. As the analyst Frida Furman observed, "Aging is largely a biologically determined phenomenon, but like any other human experience it takes place in a social world in regard to its meaning, value and significance."[2] And in this social world, as Laura Hurd wrote in the *Journal of Aging Studies*, older women are stigmatized. "Shaping the interactions and perceptions of themselves and others, the stigma associated with aging may be internalized by older women and experienced as a profound sense of shame and aversion toward their own and other older women's bodies."[3]

In the first chapter of her book *Learning to be Old*, Margaret Cruikshank makes the profound observation that aging is shaped more by culture than by biology; that is, in many ways, it is socially constructed. There is biological aging, which is inevitable, and then there is cultural aging, which is the result of the promulgation of negative beliefs. It is important to be aware of such social constructions, and it is crucial to resist them if midlife boomer women want to age comfortably: "Learning to be old," Cruikshank says, "means unlearning much of what we think is true."[4] She goes on to note that it is not the changes to our bodies that define us as old, but rather the meaning given to those changes, and is a most important marker for midlife women's roadmaps. This concept is echoed by other social commentators, who feel that aging is a biologically determined phenomenon that occurs within a socially constructed world.[5]

The major difficulty for older people, and especially women, is society's emphasis on aging as decline, replete with dreadful images of negativity and loss. This is not to say that poor health and illnesses are not real concerns. Of course they are. However, it is to say that, given the emphasis on decline, the advantages of getting older receive short shrift, and the meanings given to bodily changes are interpreted fearfully; in most instances, unnecessarily so.

Given the emphasis on the social construction of aging, at this point it is important to consider a critique that could be referred to as the "overly cultural" concept of aging. Mike Featherstone and Andrew Wernick, writing in *Images of Aging: Cultural Representations of Later Life*, state, "To highlight the importance of the body for the study of aging, then, is not to raise the spectre of biologism, the reduction of culture to the biological, nor is it to vaunt a social constructionism in which the body is conceived as a blank state on which culture can write at will."[6] In other words, they are saying that a focus on culture should not override other considerations, nor should we assume that our minds are blank slates upon which anyone can write anything. As Frida Furman has said, women are not "cultural dopes." The reality is that most women age well, are energetic, in reasonably good health, and living full lives : a view that too often gets ignored. I also want to make it clear that damaging beliefs can and should be unlearned.

Historical and Hysterical

Considering how medical and health practices developed over the years does not only help our understanding, but can be quite amusing. *For Her Own Good*, published in 1978 by Barbara Ehrenreich and Deidre English, became a landmark publication. In it, the authors trace the role of women both as patients and as lay healers before medicine became defined as a male profession and enterprise.[7] Discussing the old patriarchal order within which women lived, produced and reproduced before the development of industrialism, the authors describe women as healers, herbalists, and midwives. They were respected and even famed, having learned from their mothers and grandmothers the skills associated with raising children, healing common illnesses, and nursing the sick.

With the transformation to market economics, "The conflict between women's traditional wisdom and male expertise centred on the right to heal." Further, in the 19th century "The historical antagonist of the female lay healer was the male professional."[8] Unfortunately, the conflict in Europe took the "particularly savage form" of witch-hunting.[9] Under this guise, female healers and other older women were hunted down and executed. This, of course, also occurred in the United States. Ehrenreich and English cite the contempt of one aging female North American healer: "There! I can tell you there's win'rows o' young doctors, bilin' over with book-larnin', that is truly ignorant of what to do for the sick, and how to p'int out those paths that well people foller towards sickness. Book fools I call 'em, them young men."[10]

With the transformation from lay healing to professional medicine and the commodification of illness, female healers clearly lost out. In Victorian times and later, the medical profession consolidated its monopoly over healing by establishing a category of illness referred to as "nervous disorders," to which women were prone by nature, they being weak, dependent and diseased.[11] The "cult of female invalidism" that affected middle and upper-class women developed in the late 19th century and was a precursor of the types of syndromes discussed above. As Ehrenreich and English dryly note, many women were probably using "female invalidism" as a way to escape their reproductive and domestic duties since contraception was unreliable, and abortions were illegal. "So female invalidism may be a direct ancestor of the nocturnal 'headache' which so plagued husbands in the mid-twentieth century." Of course, after that, the advent of the pill allowed women more sexual freedom.

In a chapter entitled "Subverting the Sick Role: Hysteria,"[12] Ehrenreich and English discuss how male medical professionals decided that there was a connection between the uterus and the brain ("uterus" comes from the Greek *hyster*), the idea being that a portion of the uterus somehow detaches itself and makes its way to the brain, resulting in hysterical "fits." And according to Elizabeth Markson, writing in *The Handbook of Women and Aging*, "Not only did doctors perform hysterectomies in an attempt to cure 'hysteria', but they also held that aging women were adversely influenced by menopause."[13] Some doctors also felt that women suffered from "involutional melancholia" and "climacteric insanity."

Early in the 20th century a new type of therapy, known as psychoanalysis, ushered in by Sigmund Freud and his colleagues, became the home for (chiefly male) experts or those who considered themselves to be experts on women's lives. Depression was established as a major illness, for which modern medical science and mental health practitioners now treat both women and men. Beginning in the 1950s, anti-depressant prescriptions became, by far, the most common prescription written for women. Hysterectomies were also extravagantly performed in the latter half of the 20th century, and one wonders if women who had their uterus removed were then considered to be brainless as well. The term "hysterical woman" quickly came into popular everyday usage. There was even an episode of the TV series *All in the Family* in which Archie decided that Edith, who was suddenly and uncharacteristically standing up to him, must be going through the "change" and recommended that she visit a "groinocologist." Throughout most of the 20th century, many doctors would continue to view menstruation, pregnancy, and menopause as physical and intellectual liabilities.

The Aging Enterprise

Once the commodification of medical practices occurred, the view of aging as decline became established, and the medicalization of old age – that is, treating old age as a disease – quickly followed.

Describing this process with respect to women, the Boston Women's Health Collective comments: "The most striking example of this process is the medicalization of women's lives in all areas of reproductive health, sexuality and aging."[14] And according to Margaret Cruikshank, "the business of the old is to be sick"; she follows up by observing that this is even truer today then ever before, thanks to the increasingly large role that corporate health care plays in aging.[15] Along the same lines, Carol Estes, a respected American social policy analyst, talks about how the social construction of aging is based on a medical model which looks at the complexity of aging as a purely medical problem. And, of course, it follows that treating old age as a disease entails the intervention of a medical practitioner.[16]

Thus, what has come to be referred to as the "aging enterprise" has grown into what Estes and others have named the "medical industrial complex." This refers to the health industry in the United States, which is made up of multibillion-dollar enterprises that include doctors, hospitals, nursing homes, insurance companies and drug manufacturers.[17]

Though Canada's public health system is thankfully much different than that of the United States, a number of these observations still apply here as well. Giant pharmaceutical corporations and the media dovetail in projecting views that are seen and read by Canadian viewers and readers. Pharmaceutical corporations pitch directly to doctors through advertisements, in medical journals, and – in many cases – through gifts. Although direct-to-consumer drug advertising is not allowed in Canada, thanks to the ready availability of American TV channels, there is considerable spillover. TV ads influence middle-aged and older viewers by implanting the idea that they "need" certain drugs in order to treat a particular illness, real or imagined. The viewers, in turn, demand prescriptions for the drug from physicians, who may have received largesse from pharmaceutical representatives to encourage them to prescribe it. But it is telling that the voice-over disclaimers on TV describing possible side effects of the drug being promoted are frequently as long as the ads themselves. This alone should give pause to anyone contemplating such usage without adequate investigation.

The origins of certain so-called "syndromes" are at best highly dubious. For example, consider something called the "Hurried Woman's Syndrome," discovered by Texas physician and gynecologist Brent Bost. The symptoms of this syndrome are fatigue, low sex drive, and weight gain, with the latter leading to stress, low self-esteem, and guilt. According to Bost, some fifty million American women between the ages of twenty-five and fifty-five are affected annually. He calls it a form of pre-depression. It is hard not to agree with the critic of Bost, who, in the same report, refers to this "syndrome" as another of the "flavour of the week disorders, an example of psychologizing problems that used to be just thought of as vicissitudes of life."[18]

With all due respect to Dr. Bost, he is apparently unaware that most women have always multitasked, both in the home and outside it, and that they have always commonly and understandably felt fatigued and stressed. The surprise would be if they did not.

There is even a word for it (for those who are mothers): "Supermom." There is also the syndrome known as female sexual arousal disorder (FSAD), undoubtedly a close cousin of the Hurried Woman.

And in an article in the *Vancouver Sun*, Daphne Branham similarly refers to statistics that declare yet another "epidemic": "So now shyness is a widespsread debilitating disease afflicting us? . . . Some experts figure drug companies are manufacturing 'disorders.' Symptoms include rapid heartbeat, sweating, shaking, and an upset stomach or 'butterflies.'"[19] Who has not had such "symptoms" when waiting to write an exam, or to get the results of a worrisome medical test, or before going into a job interview? It is important to recognize that for some people such experiences can be so extreme that they do require professional assistance. However, the greater concern is that hearing what is a common reaction to everyday stressful situations being referred to as a "syndrome" can suggest that something is wrong and that help is required – probably in the form of a drug – when in fact nothing is amiss.

This issue has been discussed in *Selling Sickness* by two Canadian authors, Ray Moynihan and Alan Cassels[20], and their subtitle outlines the major issue: *How the World's Biggest Pharmaceutical Companies Are Turning Us All into Patients*. They believe that the pharmaceutical industry is working to define and design the latest disorders and dysfunctions in order to create and expand markets for their newest medicines. "Too often the aim is to turn healthy people into patients."[21] The authors cite the then Chief Executive Officer of Merck, Henry Gadsden, who some thirty years ago said it was long his dream to make drugs for healthy people. Three decades later, his dream has come true. "The ups and downs of daily life have become mental disorders, common complaints are transformed into frightening conditions, and more and more ordinary people are turned into patients."[22] Moynihan and Cassels note that not only are drug companies making what they call celebrity brands (Prozac, Viagara, and Celebrex), but increasingly they are making the diseases that go with them. Thus, more and more often we see huge pharmaceutical enterprises manufacturing both new illnesses and the drugs that can treat them, a highly profitable process.

Susan A. McDaniel, a prominent Canadian sociologist, says that "aging itself is being pathologized, requiring aggressive correctives that, of course, offer new niche markets for drug companies."[23] So what about the idea that aging is somehow preventable? Now there are new "anti-aging medicines," reminiscent of the pursuit of agelessness already discussed, which Martha Holstein describes as a "potential new weapon in the postmodern task of self-creation." Furthermore, she says, "short of a major cultural upheaval, older women will experience the negative effects of anti-aging medicine more forcefully than will men." And she goes on to point out that "women's bodies have historically been 'medicalized,' that is, treated as if normal conditions were pathological, requiring medical intervention and placed under the control of men."[24] The advent of anti-aging medicine, which includes shots of human growth hormone, or telomerase, appears to be a new form of ageism (the dislike of growing old or being old or older persons) which ignores some root causes of poor health, such as poverty, working too long and too hard, environmental degradation, and/or constant stress.[25] Another concern about anti-aging medicine is expressed by Dr. Maxwell J. Mehlman and his associates, in an article called *Anti-Aging Medicine: Can Consumers Be Better Protected?* It is their belief that such interventions are proliferating. "Some of these interventions can seriously harm older persons and aging baby boomers who consume them."[26] They see the Internet as playing an increasing role with such websites as "Youngevity: The Anti-Aging Company," and they urge health and other groups concerned with health care to take the lead in fighting the proliferation of these anti-aging medicines.

Further concerns are expressed regarding anti-aging medicines, which are felt to be an anti-aging industry, and thought to be worth some $30 billion in 2001. King and Calasanti, in their assessment of the current emphasis on individual solutions, note the formation of an anti-aging industry, including anti-aging medicine. They describe this as "a medical specialty founded on the application of advanced scientific and medical technologies for the early detection, prevention, treatment and reversal, of age-related dysfunction, disorders and diseases."[27] The American Academy of Anti-Aging Medicine (A4M) is a non-commercial, not-for-profit volunteer society of physicians and scientists who, as King and Calasanti see it, "provide the professional legitimacy for much of the anti-aging industry whose purveyors liberally avail themselves of A4M's scientific claims that aging can be halted or even reversed." Strong anti-aging medicine indeed, which many boomers may find hard to resist: science in partnership with Peter Pan.

Information regarding drug regulatory processes in Canada is insufficient. Experts interviewed for a study of the drug regulatory process in this country expressed the view that there is a need for greater transparency, and that Health Canada needs to release a lot more information to enable researchers to spot the serious health concerns posed by some prescription drugs.[28]

These are sobering insights for mid-life and older women who, searching for ways to stay youthful, may allow themselves to be seduced into "Youngevity" interventions. Perhaps, in addition to our concern over "pathologization" and "medicalization" of old age, another word, "pharmacologization," should be added to the mix.

From Menopause to Menopower

Happily, menopause is no longer considered to be "climacteric insanity," although discussing it remains a veritable minefield, given the confusions and contradictions that surround it. For example, some years back it became popular to believe that taking Vitamin E, an antioxidant, would relieve some menopausal symptoms. More recent studies find that its use is of minimal benefit.[29] Similar confusion faces pre-menopausal and menopausal women who must make important decisions about their menopausal symptoms.

While there is no shortage of information regarding approaches to menopause, the analysis by Joan Callahan in her article *Menopause: Taking the Cures or Curing the Takes?*[30] is comprehensive, focused and provides a substantive overview of the issues. Callahan outlines several ideas about menopause, one being that womanhood itself is disrupted by menopause, another that menopause is a disease in need of medical intervention. She discusses these as the "received view" on women's aging, and shows how they construct menopause as a malady. In fact, menopause involves normal endocrinal and physiological changes, and the permanent cessation of menstruation resulting from loss of ovarian follicular activity. It is a transition period of indefinite duration – commonly three to six years – during which a woman moves into a new physiological life phase, which includes the cessation of ovulation and the lowering of hormonal levels. Among other changes, it is marked by hot flashes that can be extreme in some women and mild or non-existent in others.

Callahan, who objects to the degrading cultural representations of older women, states that processes that are perfectly normal for women are constantly being medicalized. Just as pregnancy and childbirth have long been moved from the personal realm to the realm of professional medicine, as the baby boomers move into their fifties, menopause is increasingly billed as a malady requiring medical intervention.[31]

She recognizes and deplores the fact that the pharmaceutical industry has become deeply invested in the medicalization of menopause, advertising ways to "treat it," and pressing women to seek medical help.

She cites Dr. Susan Love's well-known *Hormone Book*, which explains how menopause has become big business, and how, as a result, there has been a complete flip-flop in the attitude of the medical professional towards it.[32] The profession has gone from "It's all in your head" (remember hysterical women?) to "we've got a drug for whatever symptom you might be experiencing."

Moving on to the hormone replacement therapy (HRT) debate, Callahan states that she prefers the term exogenous hormone intervention (EHI), which correctly implies estrogen coming from outside the body rather than being produced by it, because the term HRT plays into the construction of menopause as a deficiency and a disease.

In a detailed description of the many changes that occur during menopause, she notes what some of the more distressing symptoms are but thinks it important that these experiences vary *significantly* (her emphasis) from woman to woman.

Carefully examining the pros and cons of EHI with regard to cardiovascular disease, osteoporosis, and cholesterol, she concludes EHI is effective in relieving the effects of hormonal change and that short-term use is both appropriate and helpful.

However, when it comes to long-term use, this is "a more worrisome matter" as it entails serious risk of breast and endometrial cancer.[32] This is an issue that is widely discussed, with information readily available.

Once again, pre-menopausal and menopausal women are faced with a troublesome double bind: HRT (to disengage from Callahan and revert to the more popular usage) undoubtedly helps to alleviate distressing symptoms, but at what cost? A woman must decide upon short-term or long-term usage or, indeed, whether to give it a miss altogether.

Physicians themselves no doubt respond differently to the conflicting theories on HRT. The range of advice is illustrated by the following anecdotes.

One woman told this story about a visit to her physician: "I explained everything as clearly as I could, and went over my general healthy condition . . . She never once looked me in the eye – too busy writing – and all of a sudden she gave me this prescription for hormones (which I had never taken) and said, 'You should be taking estrogen' . . . I didn't have the nerve to ask her why, without a checkup and in the absence of any real reasons, I should now go on this drug."[34] In another instance, a well-informed fifty-something boomer woman explained how she had told her doctor that she was confused by the many different opinions surrounding medical approaches to menopause. Her physician quite honestly expressed his own confusions, following which they had a discussion regarding her options.

To add to the "menopause brouhaha" as the late Betty Friedan called it, a fairly recent approach to the dilemmas and decisions that menopausal women must consider is a new one called bioidentical hormones. In her book *Ageless*, author Suzanne Somers argues in favor of using bioidentical hormone replacement, claiming that unlike the estrogen pill Premarin, (made from pregnant mare's urine) bioidentical hormone replacement, being made of soy, wild yam, and other plant extracts, is therefore "drug free."[35] It's an approach that seems to be the centre of yet another debate. In an article in the *Globe and Mail* by Leah McLaren and headlined "Chrissy Snow – health guru?" Dr. Marla Shapiro, a woman's health specialist, is quoted as saying that using these ingredients doesn't make it natural.[36] "A drug is any biological substance, synthetic or non-synthetic, that is taken for non-dietary needs." Several doctors are quoted in the article as being highly skeptical, while in the book itself, Somers cites doctors who are in favour of bioidentical hormone replacement. As well, some of Somers' respondents who use these replacements swear by them.

Again, midlife women who are contemplating its use are faced with an important decision. Other women rely on alternative health practices, including herbs, vitamins, exercises, yoga, and so forth. It goes without saying that women should have regular medical checkups, including pap smears, breast examination and mammograms, although some controversy exists about having the latter for women in their forties.

Decisions need to be made on an informed basis. Women need to talk with other women, partners, physicians and other health practitioners. One very promising development is the establishment of community-based menopause clinics. These are staffed by knowledgeable advisers and offer a place where women can meet in discussion groups, ask questions, and share experiences. In communities where there aren't such clinics, it would be a timely for some mid-life boomer women to start one. In a rural area it may difficult to do this, but a chatroom in cyberspace may be helpful. Getting information, questioning and talking to knowledgeable persons are ways in which women can exercise agency and take control of their natural bodily progressions.

Regular or Lite?

Given the degree of ageism within our culture, it is not surprising that the sex lives of older people are fodder for insulting stereotypes and ageist humor. Comedian George Burns once commented, "I'm at an age now where just putting my cigar in its holder is a thrill," and Milton Berle remarked, "Sex at the age of eighty-four is a wonderful experience – especially the one in the winter." There is also the anecdote that was related by an older woman to a younger one: "You're lucky. You don't have to worry about lying on top . . . you know. When we lean over our sag really sags."[37] Such disparaging comments about older people and later life sex may be good for laughs, but they contribute to negative views of sexuality in later life.

A number of years ago in California an older women's discussion group, composed of newly retired and about-to-retire women, was formed. Aged sixty and over, these women were unhappy about the lack of information pertaining to their needs, and one of the group's topics was sexuality and menopause. When the discussion turned to older women and sexual activities, the group expressed strong feelings that older women should continue to be sexual.[38] One woman declared that her sex life gotten much better after menopause. A few others felt that they had plenty of sex drive after menopause and that, to the degree that they were sexually active, they had good relations. A few said that they enjoyed not having to worry about pregnancy and menstruation. Some others felt that there was considerable companionship between older men and women, but were not sure that it was sexual. The discussion on later-life sexuality touched on those women in the group who were not partnered, and who felt ambivalent about their situation, wondering about both the advantages and disadvantages of being with another person. One unpartnered woman noted drolly that she wished she could meet a man who interested her as much as a baked potato.

Older women and men don't necessarily define their sexuality in terms of intercourse, so much as in terms of intimacy, which includes touching, hugging, kissing, and cuddling. There is even a name for such preferences: "outercourse." As people age, changes occur that can affect sexuality. For example, estrogen levels drop after menopause, and this can affect sexual performance. As well, health problems are an issue, since drugs taken for conditions like high blood pressure, depression, and diabetes may affect the libido. On the other hand, for some midlife and older women there may be an advantage – that of not being interrupted by work or children so that sex, if they are so inclined, can be an unhurried and pleasurable event.

In most discussions of midlife and older women, their health and sexuality, one issue that does not receive sufficient attention is that of older lesbian women. According to Susan McDaniel and Sharon Abu-Laden, "The invisibility of lesbian women generally and aging lesbian women in particular works in contradictory ways: both to conceal lesbians' experience with aging and to reinforce prevalent stereotypes about lesbians."[39] Writer Suzanne Slater, discussing health and other late-life changes that affect both lesbian and heterosexual couples, says with aging lesbian partners "the nature of the couple's emotional and physical intimacy may likewise be affected as they enter a stage of life containing difficult compromises and likely personal losses."[40] According to psychologist Olive Skene Johnson, older lesbians have a lower frequency of sex than do older straight women. She feels that this "is not surprising, considering that many women who call themselves lesbians are motivated by factors other than erotic attraction to women."[41] Cruikshank points out that "some older women who would be regarded by others as lesbians because of lifelong emotional attachments to women and an absence of heterosexual partnerships, do not identify themselves as lesbians."[42] She suggests that with the growing acceptance of gay and lesbian lifestyles, older women may "come out" as they reach their sixties and seventies. Given the homophobic environment in which gays and lesbians have spent their lives, older lesbians would be drawn to each other to fill social and other needs, especially if their families, employers and others do not accept them.

The following is a brief excerpt from a round table discussion on the topic of health in relation to gays and lesbians that was held on *50plus Online Magazine*:

50plus Magazine: You are all gay and past 50. What's on your minds these days?

Edward: Well, just like just everyone in the 50plus age group . . . gay and lesbian seniors are concerned about their health . . .The thought of relying on others for health care is very frightening because I know we have to turn to networks and social institutions that have not always been tolerant of us.

Ruth: I know what you mean. Gays and lesbians . . . still encounter negative reactions from health providers.

It is especially difficult for we seniors who grew up prior to gay liberation.

Ellen: In much of America and Canada, there is still overt discrimination by both the medical professions and the public in general. When we're looking for health care, we come up against a lot of obstacles.

George: Many gay and lesbian seniors revert back to the closet, keeping their sexual orientation hidden ... I know many people who withheld that information when they needed health care.[43]

This glimpse into the gay and lesbian community's health concerns in the context of prevailing antagonism against them also provides an example of a schism between younger and older gays and lesbians, about which straight people need to learn much more.

Recently attitudes have changed a great deal towards gay and lesbian people, thanks in good part to persistent lesbian-gay-bisexual-transgendered (LGBT) activism, which is challenging homophobic, discriminatory and legislative inequalities.

My own grandkids seem to be completely at ease with the idea of same-sex relationships, and appear to be comfortable with any gay or lesbians teachers or friends they have or have had. This could certainly not be said of the attitudes prevalent when I and others of the current generation of older women and men were young. Given changing attitudes and increasing support, it is likely that midlife and older lesbians may have an easier time than did their forebears.

To its credit, Canada, along with the Netherlands, Belgium, Spain, and South Africa have legalized same-sex marriage. However, in the United States same-sex marriage functioned as a wedge issue and was featured strongly in the religious right's backing of George W. Bush in the 2004 presidential election. Clearly there is still much to be achieved.

There are several older women who discuss sex on television. Much of this talk is explicit: one thinks of the renowned and effervescent "Dr. Ruth" Westheimer. Sue Johanson, who is about seventy years old, until recently did a weekly sex advice TV show called *Talk Sex with Sue Johanson*. Sometimes called the "sex lady," Johanson is clearly comfortable discussing sex toys and giving advice on intimate sexual questions posed by her phone-in listeners. Johansen retired recently, but continues as a consultant. A newspaper feature about her by Tony Atherton, *Sexlady Likes to Work at Home*, opened with: "It's getting to be routine for Sue Johanson. A security agent in some US airport will look at the collection of provocative shapes showing on his [sic] X-ray of her carry-on bag, and then at the wizened [sic] iron-haired woman waiting to collect it." Farther down in the article the writer describes her as "frisky," an adjective one might have thought more appropriate for a household pet, and one wonders how many readers noted this journalist's ageism and sexism. However, he does go on to say that, for almost a generation, Johanson has been helping Canadians to become more comfortable with their sexuality. With her growing celebrity in the United States, Johanson is now talking in the US as well. The picture accompanying the article is amusing, showing Johanson during a sex education talk to university students. To illustrate that "one size fits all," both arms raised overhead, she is pulling on a condom that she has stretched to about three feet in length.[44] Johansen retired recently, but continues as a consultant. In addition, a recent documentary entitled *Still Doing It* focuses on the sexual lives of nine women aged between sixty-seven and eighty-seven. One of the women in the documentary comments: "Sexuality is not an off/on switch. It's a dimmer switch that each couple needs to set at the right level for them. It might not be set as bright as it once was, but it can still provide a warm intimate glow."[45]

Illness, Wellness, and Fitness

The other side of the longevity coin is that as mid-life boomer women get older, they may have to deal with chronic illness, but this is not necessarily a calamity.

In fact, the large majority of Canadian women living at home – that is, who are non-institutionalized – describe their general health in positive terms. The proportion of women who report chronic or degenerative health problems does rise with age, of course, and that should come as no surprise, given their gains in life expectancy.

According to the Statistics Canada publication *Women in Canada - Fifth Edition*, women's health involves their emotional, social, physical and spiritual well-being. The determinants of health levels include income, social status, education, employment, and working conditions in complex inter-relatedness.[46] Biological determinants are also important, including genetic make-up. And given Canada's public health care system, which aims to provide equal access to all, I would consider social policy in relation to health to be important as well.

Some of the health conditions reported by women include non-food allergies, arthritis, high blood pressure, and recurring migraines, with smaller numbers suffering from food allergies, asthma, diabetes, or heart disease.[47] Senior women are more likely to report chronic health conditions and disabilities, particularly in the over-eighty-five age group, one of the fastest growing female age categories. Cancer and heart disease are among the leading causes of death among women.[48]

There are also gender differences in health, with women being more likely than men to report multiple health problems, and also more likely to take medications than are men, even when birth control and menopause-related drugs are excluded.[49] Women are also more likely to consult physicians. As Chappell et al say in *Aging in Contemporary Canada*, "Social acceptability due to socialization and to traditional roles may mean it is more acceptable for women than for men to adopt the sick role . . . Women discuss their health more freely than do men."[50] It appears that men have been traditionally socialized to deny experiencing symptoms of illness, thus discussing their health concerns with fewer people. This interpretation gives rise to a macho male model of experiencing illness. But contrary to arguments that, as men and women adopt more similar lifestyles, they will become more alike, the authors cite a study that found social structural factors, such as being in a high income category, working full time, caring for a family and social support, are stronger determinants of health for women, whereas for men it is personal health practices, such as smoking and alcohol consumption that are the determinants. It is their belief that women's multiple roles can result in role overload and role conflict (the double day) putting strains on their health – an analysis that is contrary to a simplistic Hurried Women's Syndrome.

Also worthy of note is Chappell et al's finding that, despite evidence to the contrary, the belief persists that mental well-being decreases with age. They feel that, though physical health declines, psychological health increases, an encouraging concept for mid-life women, as it is counter to the standard decline-as-we-age thesis. However, it would surprise no one that some older women, particularly those who are single, isolated, and struggling to make ends meet, would be depressed. In the authors' words, "The determinants of health, including health beliefs, health behaviors and the social structure, influence our health . . ."[51] They also feel that such determinants are all relatively new areas of study, and that governments and community groups can, in fact, effect change.

Turning from illness to fitness, if there is substance to the general belief that baby boomers have changed every aspect of their lives as they reach various stages, their interest in fitness is way out front. According to Dr. Arlene Bierman, the author of *Aging Well: What Every Woman Should Know*, the fountain of youth can not be found at the tip of a Botox-filled syringe, but rather in physical activity.[52] Dr. Richard Levandowski echoes this approach in an article titled "The Anti-Aging Combo: fitness, flexibility.": "While certain aspects of aging are inevitable, there are signs associated with aging that can be avoided, even reversed, with physical activity. This is great news especially for the first of some 75 million American baby boomers who are turning 60 this year."[53] The advanced cohort of Canada's more than nine million baby boomers turned sixty in 2006.

A comprehensive, recent Canadian research study on baby boomers and their health dynamics conducted by Canadian gerontologist Dr. Andrew V. Wister – the author of *Baby Boomer Health Dynamics: How Are We Aging?* – provides solid research and a gendered analysis of the fitness phenomenon.[54] Discussing the complexities of healthy individual and population lifestyles, he notes: "There has been speculation as to whether baby boomers are faring as well as mid-life persons of the same age a generation ago (e.g. in the 1970s) in terms of lifestyle and health."[55] In his examination of this question he found that while "unhealthy exercise levels" – meaning exercise levels below recommended guidelines – have declined over the period of his study (the twenty-two years from 1978/79 to 2000/1), it was more pronounced among baby boomers in 2000/1 compared to persons of the same age in 1978/79. Measures include persons reporting exercise levels that are below the recommended guidelines, that is, less than three exercise intervals a week of at least fifteen to twenty minutes each. Activity includes brisk walking, jogging, racket sports, weight training, and exercises. Therefore, while boomers are embracing an active lifestyle to a greater extent, there is considerable room for improvement. In other words, baby boomers are exercising more, but not enough to meet recommended guidelines, and are not reaping the full benefits of active lifestyles. This certainly sheds surprising light with respect to the common belief that Canadian baby boomers are model exercisers. Here are some baby boomer health factors that Wister analyzed, including other eye-openers:

- *Smoking*. There has been a decline in rates of smoking for both men and women. Baby boomers smoking rates were 40.4% lower among persons thirty five to fifty-four from 1978/9 to 2000/1.

- *Heavy drinking*. A wide gender gap persists. For males aged fifteen and over, drinking declined from 21.8% in 1978/9 to 10.1% in 2000/1. For females, the drop was from 7% in 1978/79 to 3.1% in 2000/01. Baby boomers drink less then their counterparts a generation ago: in 2000/1, 6.3% of persons aged thirty-five to fifty-four were drinking heavily compared to 13.8% in 1978/79.

- *Boomer Obesity*: A Bulging Bulge. The author asserts that great concern is in order with respect to body mass index (BMI) among baby boomers.

He found an upward pattern of obesity across the lifespan – in fact, a doubling of the obesity rate for both men and women – and calls this "a shocking trend.'" For males aged twenty to sixty-four, obesity jumped from 7.1% in 1985 to 16.3% in 2000/01; for females, the rate nearly tripled from 5.8% to 14.2%. The rate for baby boomers in 2000/1 aged thirty-five to fifty-four was 16%, compared to about half that rate of 8.2% in 1985.[56]

Wister found the consumption of soft drinks in the US doubled between 1975 and 1997, from about sixty litres per person to one-hundred-six litres per year. There has also been a rise in the number of oils and fats consumed. Eating outside the home has become more commonplace, along with super-sized portions, with the fast food industry leading the way. Some examples are: McDonald's French fries servings were about two ounces in the 1950s, and they are now five ounces; hamburgers have grown from about one ounce to between four and ten ounces; and soft drink sizes have doubled or tripled in volume. Even muffins, bagels, and other grain products have been super-sized. Carbonated soft drinks at fast food restaurants have swelled from eight ounces in the late 1950s to twelve ounces for a child's drink and thity-two ounces for a large adult drink.[57] Wister refers to this as an "exercise-obesity paradox," – more food than needed is eaten, while at the same time boomers are under-exercising.

Given the super-sized and incessant advertising aimed at younger and younger children, in addition to those aimed at teenagers – who are depicted as "cool" if they are devouring a bathtub-sized drink or popping some nutritionally deprived concoction into the toaster – in conjunction with the numbers of harassed mothers working outside the home who are short of time and harangued by their children to go to fast-food outlets, it should come as no surprise that there is an unhealthy gain in weight.

Low-income families, including those headed by single mothers, are hard-pressed to resist lower-priced meals at fast food outlets, especially at the end of the month when resources are dwindling. As a result, more and more children are suffering from diabetes and hypertension: yet another frightening development. This phenomenon is being globalized, with a rise in obesity even in China (perhaps since McDonalds was established there). Wherever fast foods go, fat is sure to follow. Shocking, indeed.

Women and Disability: A Slow Dance

The worlds of older disabled women and disabled women in general appear to be neglected, and as Jenny Morris has written in *Encounters with Strangers*, this neglect includes even those who are interested in women's issues. Commenting on this exclusion, Morris points out the concerns that are at the centre of non-disabled women's lives are the same ones that are relevant to disabled women. She feels that this exclusion renders feminist theory incomplete, as it makes no attempt to understand the interaction between the social construct of gender and the social construct of disability. She give an example of similarity with abled women in the case of single women parents who generally face questions about their abilities to raise children alone; such questions are also directed at disabled single women parents, but with the addition of discriminatory attitudes towards their disability.[58]

In Canada, women make up the majority of the Canadian population with disabilities. In 2001, 54% of those who had a disability were women, whereas females accounted for only 54% of the total population. The likelihood of women having disabilities also increases with age. In 2001, 42% of all women aged sixty-five and over had a disability, almost twice the figure among women aged fifty-five to sixty-four. The largest proportion of women with disabilities have a mild disability, but 14% of women aged fifteen and over with disabilities had a severe disability.[59]

According to Sue Wendell's landmark book, *The Rejected Body: Feminist Philosophical Reflections on Disability*, a definition of disability is complicated, and different definitions have different outcomes. "Definitions of disability officially accepted by government bureaucracies and social service agencies determine people's legal and practical entitlements to many forms of assistance."[60] These may include getting help for education or training, obtaining equipment such as wheelchairs and computers, modifying a home, hiring assistants, or getting transportation. As Wendell points out, "Recognition of a person's disability by the people s/he is closest to is important not only for receiving their help . . . but for receiving the acknowledgement and confirmation of her/his reality, so essential for keeping a person socially and psychologically anchored in a community."[61] Hence, according to this expert, the importance of having a definition. Unless a formal diagnosis is made, Wendell feels it is not uncommon for friends and family members to write off someone's symptoms as mere "aches and pains."

One older disability activist is Bonnie Sherr Klein, the noted Canadian filmmaker and author of *Slow Dance: A Story of Stroke, Love and Disability*.[62] Now disabled herself, she is currently an activist in the disability arts movement and her latest National Film Board film, '*SHAMLESS: The Art of Disability*' was released in 2006. I have learned a great deal through my friendship with Bonnie and now look upon the world with very different eyes than I did before I met her.

For example, I am now keenly aware of whether a building or a movie theatre is accessible to disabled persons, or whether curbs can be navigated by someone in a wheelchair or a scooter. Thankfully, progress is being made with regard to recognizing the need to make public spaces amenable to the disabled community. But there are deeper problems as well, some of which are touched on in the following interview I conducted with Bonnie.

Zimmerman: What health problems are particular to older disabled women?

Klein: Unfortunately, this is a topic that hasn't been studied adequately. Research was done by D.A.W.N. The DisAbled Women's Network, but funding costs have limited their ability. There is a women's disability network, but there is a lack of knowledge in general. One of the most important factors in dealing with or accommodating disability is having personal networks. The networks of friendships nurture people with disabilities.

Zimmerman: Are you aware of any effects on older disabled women's health?

Klein: Until now many disabilities, for example quadriplegia, limited people's lifespans. Any evidence of longer life spans is because medical practice in general has improved, but there is less information on this because disabled women haven't lived long enough.

Zimmerman: What are the different categories of disability?

Klein: Basically the categories are physical, sensory, and intellectual disabilities and mental health. People who have survived strokes and some other illnesses, who have speech impairment like asphasia or memory impairment are mistaken for those who are intellectually handicapped.

Zimmerman: But some disabilities are those that a person is born with?

Klein: Yes, some one is born with, others [are] acquired. Mine is acquired, the result of a brain injury that left me with disabilities. This event parachuted me into early old age, [giving me] a preview of problems older people experience, which includes reduced mobility, severe fatigue, lack of energy, and some cognitive loss.

Zimmerman: Could you explain what you mean by "cognitive loss"?

Klein: Well, there is a diminished ability to classify and organize things. I am better doing one thing at a time. As my late mother-in-law aged, she became impatient with doing one thing at a time. Because of this I feel a real affinity with older people, and they in turn, have an affinity with me. This is very leveling from the perspective of class privilege. I feel a sense in which like everyone else, I have a sense of oneness in terms of human vulnerability.

Words from the wise.

Gender Benders

Some years ago, a woman in her late sixties found herself with a health problem, which – while not major – was troublesome. She consulted her family physician, a man who was aware of ageism among some medical practitioners and prided himself on being knowledgeable about New Age issues. The woman was also in transition, becoming more assertive as she moved away from the mainly passive and unquestioning attitudes of her generation. Her medical problem proved to be stubborn and as both of them – he as a physician and she as a patient – became more frustrated, each regressed to their former roles: he became more authoritarian, she became more passive. The woman in this anecdote is me, and the lesson learned was that reconstructing culturally prescribed roles is not easy, particularly within certain contexts.

The interaction described above, however, may be representative of the type of encounters that will occur as physicians and other health practitioners face increasing numbers of mid-life and older women. Many older women have been socialized to accept their (mainly male) physicians' advice with unquestioning deference. His – and in some cases her – authority was seldom challenged, even though he/she may be overtly ageist and/or sexist. One immediately thinks of the abhorrent exposes of male physicians sexually abusing their female patients, but ageism is more likely to appear in such comments as, "Well, what can you expect at your age?" This type of comment is reinforced by older patients who say things like "I guess I have to expect these things to happen at my age," thus encouraging passivity. There is an old joke about a ninety-year-old woman who goes to her physician to complain about a sore left knee. When the doctor's response is of the well-what-can-you-expect-at-your-age variety, she replies that her right knee is the same age as her left one and it is quite all right. The point is that such attitudes within the doctor/patient relationship coincide with the cultural assumption that getting older means decline.

One possible result of this complacency could well be that a symptom needing treatment could be overlooked. An American study conducted by Jon F. Nussbaum et al and entitled *Ageism and Ageist Language Across the Life Span* found that general internists and family physicians tend to display an unwillingness to provide primary care services to the elderly population, preferring to treat younger, healthier patients.[63] They note that this may be in part because of the complexities of dealing with the American medicare system (or the lack thereof). The authors also found that ageism, especially in the form of negative stereotypes of older patients, is of special concern with regard to attitudes towards women. One of the most unwanted results of such attitudes is that some women end up having only limited involvement in decisions relating to their care. Physicians also tend to dismiss older women's complaints of such things as incontinence and arthritis as part of normal aging. Nussbaum and his colleagues are particularly critical about the use of patronizing and condescending language, which affects more women patients than men. In their discussion of ageist attitudes expressed through language, they cite staff in long-term care facilities using "patronizing speech in the form of baby talk."[64] Most of these staff persons felt that such usage is all right, and even welcomed. The authors feel that imposing such child-like qualities might create dependency in older women. I was astounded when I read this, and tried to imagine a reverse scenario where I would talk authoritatively to a nurse or physician who would then answer me in baby talk. As the saying goes, it boggles the mind.

The topic of the gender of doctors and their female patients was discussed in one of the focus groups I organized when preparing this book. There was a mixed response to the idea that women physicians showed more sensitivity to mid-life or older women than did male physicians. One of the older women, who had been accompanied by her daughter when she went to see a female physician, found that the doctor addressed all her comments to her daughter "as if I wasn't there." Another woman, however, stated that she "preferred women physicians because they are much more aware of women's illness, and don't cut you off." Still another commented, "A male doctor I had treated me like a dummy and hurried me." These anecdotes are far from definitive, yet it is possible that if more women were asked the same question, there might be a similar range of responses. However, with changes swirling around us and the increasing unacceptability of ageist and sexist practices, boomer women may not long tolerate negative attitudes, implied or otherwise. A recent excellent study notes that "female physicians are changing the day-to-day practice of medicine, emphasizing collaboration over compliance in decision-making about women's health issues."[65] A female surgeon I interviewed, herself a baby boomer, told me that she involves her patients in all decision-making, no matter what their age. And several baby boom women professionals I know, including my own daughters, tell me that they definitely participate in any decision-making regarding their health.

It is interesting to consider how these issues are playing out within current training. In Canada, the growth in the numbers of women enrolled in medicine has grown hugely. Recent Canadian medical school classes have a range of 43%-74% women (mean 58%) compared to the range for men of 26%-57% (mean 42%).[66] Thus, it is crucial that medical faculties in this country rid their curricula of any ageist or sexist attitudes. Recognizing the many societal changes that medical practitioners are presently addressing, or will be addressing in the near future, the Faculty of Medicine at the University of Ottawa has established an office of Equity, Diversity and Gender Issues, which follows these three major principles. This is a highly commendable model for present and future medical practitioners.[67]

That there is a pressing need for changes in attitudes by some health practitioners towards older people, particularly with regard to older women, is emphasized by what is described as a disturbing new Canadian study. A study of 466,792 adult patients admitted to thirteen Ontario hospitals between Jan 1, 2001 and Dec. 31, 2002 showed that older women with heart failure and other critical conditions receive less life support, and die more often than men in Intensive Care Units. The study conducted at the University of Toronto found "Among older patients being female was associated with a 20% increased risk of death in ICU, an eight% increased risk of death in hospital and a six-percent increased risk of death over one year."[68] I find it acceptable to refer to this ground-breaking study as both shocking and frightening. These findings tell us that older women have less chance of staying alive in certain critical illness situation than have older men- and this at the hands of medical practitioners, recognizing of course that the researchers themselves are practitioners. Can any boomer reading this think of how absolutely unacceptable this would be if it described a racial or ethnic population, rather than an ageist and sexist one? Any boomer women or men caring for elderly relatives should mark this as a health roadblock on their roadmaps.

It is to be hoped that such an enlightened outlook permeates other medical faculties across the country. In this way, some of the problems expressed by my focus group women could be alleviated by the next generation of medical graduates sensitive to both ageism and sexism.

Vital Signs

Canada's public health care system is one of the finest among industrialized nations, and to date Canadians continue to support this enviable egalitarian system that was designed "to ensure that all eligible residents of Canada have reasonable access to medically necessary insured services on a prepaid basis without direct charges at the point of service for such sections."[69] The Canada Health Act (CHA) is governed by five major principles: public administration, comprehensiveness, universality, portability and accessibility. In fact, Canadians consider their health care system to be a basic value inseparable from their national identity. It is so important to Canadians that it was a major plank in the recent Federal Elections.

At present, however, a serious debate is taking place in the country between those who insist that Canada retain its enviable egalitarian system of care, and those who wish to privatize aspects of the system, making certain procedures more easily available to those who can afford them. The system is under attack "for inefficiency, insufficient funding, and failure to meet some patients' needs in a timely fashion."[70] Midlife women, now entering a time of life when illness may require medical and professional assistance while at the same time they are dealing with aging parents and their medical problems, have a vested interest in the maintenance of a public system as do all older Canadians. Robert Steinbrook, writing in the *New England Journal of Medicine*, outlines the debate succinctly: on the one hand he cites an orthopedic surgeon who feels that significant reform is needed and that an increase in private health care will benefit the public system; on the other hand, he cites a medical spokesperson who opposes both privatization of care delivery and a parallel private system of financing care. It is the latter's opinion that a lot of money can be made by breaking medicare, and that an increase in private care will undermine the public system.[71] Those who support privatization claim that long wait times – one of the chief inefficiencies within the public system – may be averted by users going to private servers and paying for the privilege. This could constitute a "second tier system," one tier for those using the public system and the other for those with the ability to jump the queue by paying fees.

To add to the mix is the fact that under the Canadian constitution, the federal government has primary responsibility for taxation, but the provinces have primary responsibility for managing health care. As Steinbrook writes, "This leads to frequent skirmishes between the two levels of government."[72]

The Canadian system as presently constituted is a mix of both the private and public sector, 70% being public with the remainder private. Small wonder that there is confusion and a proliferation of points of view.

Basically, privately funded medical services aim to make a profit for shareholders; that is, they are based on the commodification of health and other medical goods and services. If the criterion for medical access is based on the ability of the more affluent to pay private fees, then the complexion and principles of the CHA will have to change. It will move from accessibility to all citizens (regardless of income, age and so on) to those who can afford it. As Chappell et al point out in *Aging in Contemporary Canada*, "Privatization has implications in terms of diminished control by citizens through government and increased control by business interests of multinationals over the health of Canadians."[73] Health care as we have seen, is a multi-billion-dollar corporate enterprise, especially in the United States which does not have a universal system of public health care, except for those with very low income (Medicaid) and for those over sixty-five (Medicare). Not surprisingly, given the increased for-profit ideology and business-oriented health care systems in the United States, by the end of the 1990s, private insurers and others were looking to Canada to expand their investment and were demanding greater freedom to deliver health care here under the terms of the North America Free Trade Agreement (NAFTA).[74] One result of the American system, according to a

Harvard study, is that nearly half of all personal bankruptcies in the United States are triggered by medical bills racked up due to serious illnesses or accidents. In addition, the study found that even people who had health insurance through their employers were being forced to declare bankruptcy in an effort to escape overwhelming debts. In fact, about 75% of those who said that medical bills had triggered their bankruptcy had insurance coverage at the beginning of their illnesses. For some, the insurance either lapsed or did not cover their needs.[75] Approximately forty-three million Americans have no health insurance at all. This is clear evidence of the high personal and financial costs of maintaining a non-universal health system, which is to date outside the Canadian experience.

There is no doubt that given population aging and the fact that the frail elderly become more dependent on health care – especially those over eighty-five, the majority of whom are women – health care in Canada has to meet major challenges. In addition, the advance of medical technology, though it brings great benefits, is a mixed blessing because it is expensive. In the interests of cost-saving, "restructuring" has occurred in some provinces, including the closing of hospital beds, the delisting of such services as eye exams, podiatry, chiropractic and massage therapy. Home care has also suffered cuts. This is at a time, according to Roy

Romanow's discussion paper, *Homecare in Canada*, when the need increases daily and presently exists under a patchwork of service delivery.[76] Today, when possible, short surgeries are conducted on an outpatient basis, which, in fact, is an improvement. Whether directly or indirectly as a result of such reforms and in conjunction with an aging population, waiting lists have become longer and people awaiting surgeries are understandably angry.

The media, through selection of issues and points of view and constant repetition that generally plays up the weaknesses in the system, helps create a growing dissatisfaction with the Canadian health system.

However, in 2006 when a private "Urgent Care Clinic" opened in BC-such clinics have been sardonically labeled "health care boutiques" – an exception to mainstream health reporting, Canadian medical journalist Andre Picard wrote, "While tales of interminable waiting are legion . . . with horrific stories about visits to Emergency Rooms . . . the median waiting time is 51 minutes. One in 10 patients waits less than five minutes, and one in 10 patients waits more than three hours." Picard notes that the teeth gnashing for those people enduring long waits is caused in part because a full Emergency Room has to wait for beds for trauma patients.[77] This, of course, could be a consequence of the closing of beds in some hospitals.

Two things should be emphasized when looking at the Canadian health care system: drug costs and population aging. Michael Mendelson and Pamela Divinsky point out in *Globalization and the Future of Canada's Health Care* that "drugs are the fastest growing cost in the total Canadian health-care budget." However, it is true that the price of drugs is lower here than in the US. In fact, American seniors who can't afford the high price of drugs in their country have come to Canada by the busload to get prescriptions filled or buy Canadian drugs on the internet. Some of them report that they are unable to afford their medications, sometimes cutting the dosage in half, sometimes simply doing without. One rather black-humored and true story was told to me about an older American couple faced with high prescription costs for the long-ailing husband. One day the wife arrived home, having just bought yet another prescription for about US$200, to find her husband had died. As soon as she finished notifying everyone as required, she returned to the pharmacy to get her money back. Fortunately, Canada has a Drug Price Review Board to keep things somewhat in hand.

Many social analysts do not support the crisis view of the Canadian system. As David Cheal suggests, "Before allowing ourselves to be stampeded into an alarmist stance, it might be useful to pause and consider some alternative points of view." In a book

Cheal edited, *Aging and Demographic Change in a Canadian Context*, he goes on to "warn that exaggerated concerns about population aging, or in other words demographic fears, can be harmful to rational policy making."[79] His view is supported by other analysts. For example, examining historical health spending growth and long-term projections for true health spending, Jackson and McDermott concluded that health care in Canada will remain affordable over the next forty years as long as the economy and private spending continue to grow at a moderate pace.[80] And in regard to population aging, Mendelson and Divinsky found "The population over 75 years of age will grow from 5.8% of the total population in 2001 to 6.7% in 2016. Even if we assume that the over-75 population currently accounts for 50% of health care expenditures, or about half of the current system's 9% of GDP, the additional elderly *will add only 1.1% to health care expenditures as a percentage of GDP*" (Emphasis added).[81]

Others similarly feel there is little to support the repeatedly heard lament that population aging will bankrupt our health system. John Lorinc, writing "The Medicare Myth that Refuses to Die" in the *Globe and Mail*, August 9th, 2008 cites a number of Canadian experts who feel that though costs will rise, it will not be due only to boomers aging. Inflationary pressure is due to other factors, such as rising drug costs and salaries for health care providers. Seniors are healthier today, except for obesity. One of the experts cited feels that the medicare myth is a red herring promulgated by groups favouring more private care and investment.

In addition, a study presented in a new online Canadian medical journal *Open Medicine*, as reported in the *Globe and Mail* April 19, 2007, found that Canada's much maligned healthcare produces as good or better outcomes and does so at less than half the cost than in the US The US has its mix of public/ private, but principally private providers spend annually around US $7,100 per capita contrasted to US $2,900 spent in Canada.

What have all these complexities got to do with mid-life boomer women? First, they will live longer than those who came before them and may well experience chronic illness, thereby standing to gain or lose much in terms of future health care policy developments. Second, it is well-known that people with low incomes suffer disproportionately poor health, a situation that would be exacerbated by a two-tiered health system requiring payment of fees. Older women are especially prone to this, many of them being single, separated or divorced, and statistics show that women's income drops dramatically following separation or divorce. In addition, the majority of women now in mid-life could be widowed by the age of seventy-five, as is the case with women of the present older generation. Though the poverty rates of older unattached women have substantially improved in recent years, still over 37% of unattached women aged sixty-five and over live at or below the poverty line.[82] Thus, a more privatized health system would compound their difficulties.

There is another issue that will likely affect a large majority of mid-life boomer women, that is, the need to look after ailing parents. This is already occurring for some and will affect more and more boomers as they and their parents get older. This task falls largely on the family, a term that is often a euphemism for the fact that the majority of caregivers are mid-life women. In fact, in 2007, 57% of caregivers over forty-five were women, contrasted to 43% of men (see Chapters 4 & 5).

Canadian boomers were born and brought up in a time when health care was available, dependable and not under attack, and they may not readily accept the current push towards privatizing it further. They have certainly shown themselves to favour preventative health practices, such as fitness and exercise, to guard against the risks of illness, although some improvement is needed in this area. In addition, at least for those who can afford it, enlightened boomers seek good nutrition and alternative health pathways. There are ways to involve the private sector. In seeking to lessen the current conundrum regarding lengthy waiting lists, for example using private clinics for certain procedures make sense, provided that the procedures are within the public health guidelines.

Given their increasing numbers, midlife boomer women who are in the crossfire in the public/private health care wrangles could undoubtedly make strong advocates for the preservation and improvement of Canada's system. Size and gender do matter . . .

Things You Can Do As A Boomer Woman Change Agent:

- Again (and again) decline to decline. If you are attending or accompanying a parent or older woman to see a physician or other medical professional and she/he uses the what-can-you-expect-at-your-age line, tell her/him that you do not appreciate it. Or see another physician. A practitioner with a negative attitude may not pursue a symptom that may be treatable.

- Resist the "flavour of the week" syndrome. For example, it is natural to occasionally feel low during dark winter days, or in dreary weather. Most of us do feel depressed at such times, and it does not mean we have a medical condition. If depression becomes long-term, then a professional should be consulted, but otherwise resist succumbing to so-called syndromes for the ups and downs of ordinary life.

- Pass on the muffin or bagel with cream cheese that accompanies a latte or expresso or mug of coffee. They are not health foods. Ask about the fat content of the item, even if the cream cheese is listed as "lite" and voice your objections if you have any.

• Given the increasing obesity in this country, it is easy to say that you and/or your children should cut down on sedentary activities like watching TV or playing video games. A certain amount of personal discipline is required as well as rules for children restricting the hours they can watch TV. Find out what other parents are doing to be effective. And object to the increasing sale of junk food in schools. Others are now protesting. Join them.

• Canadians feel they are entitled to make a choice between the public health system and private medical enterprises, and it is their right to do so. However, for those who wish to maintain public health care, there are advocacy groups. If there isn't one in your neighborhood, try starting one with a similarly minded spouse, friend, or relative. Inform yourself of possible changes that could improve present shortcomings to the system. It is not beyond the wits of policy makers to implement changes. Public pressure is important.

• Numbers of mid-life boomers, especially women, are already taking or will have to take responsibility for caring for ailing parents and other older relatives. An appropriate national homecare program, for which a number of models exist, would go a long way toward easing the physical, mental and emotional stress for both those caregivers who are in the paid work force and those who work at home. This is especially pertinent for those who do both childcare and eldercare. Romanow's discussion paper states that a legion of homecare users and providers, advocacy groups, politicians and researchers argue that Canada needs a national homecare program. Seek them out in your community and add your voice.

References

1. Barbara Macdonald and Cynthia Rich, *Look Me in the Eye: Old Women and Ageism* (San Francisco: Spinster's Ink Books, 1984), 23.

2. Frida Kerner Furman, *Facing the Mirror: Older Women and Beauty Shop Culture* (New York and London: Routledge, 1997), 92.

3. Laura C. Hurd, "WE'RE NOT OLD: Older Women's Negotiations of Aging and Oldness," *Journal of Aging Studies* 13, 4 (1997), 422.

4. Margaret Cruikshank, *Learning to be Old: Gender, Culture and Aging* (Lanham: Roman and Littlefield Publishers, 2003), ix.

5. See for example, Furman, *Facing the Mirror*, Chap. 2; Elizabeth Markson, in Handbook on Women and Aging, ed. Jean M. Coyle (Westbrook: Greenwood Press, 1997), Ch. 5; Sara Ruddick, in *Mother Time: Women, Aging and Ethics*, ed. Margaret Urban Walker (Lantham: Roman and Littlefield Publishers, 1999), Ch. 3.

6. Mike Featherstone and Andrew Wernick, *Images of Aging: Cultural Representations of Later Life* (London and New York: Routledge, 1995), 3.

7. Barbara Ehrenreich and Deirdre English, *For Her Own Good: 150 Years of the Experts' Advice to Women* (Garden City, NY: Anchor Press/Doubleday, 1978).

8. Ibid., 30.

9. Ibid., 30.

10. Ibid., 36.

11. Ibid., 92.

12. Ibid., 120.

13. Elizabeth Markson, "Sagacious, Sinful, or Superfluous? The Social Construction of Older Women," in *Handbook of Women and Aging: Women, Aging and Ethics*, ed. Jean M. Coyle (Westport, CT and London: Greenwood Press, 1997), 60.

14. Boston Women's Health Collective, *Our Bodies, Ourselves: For the New Century* (New York: Touchtone, 1998), 684.

15. Cruikshank, *Learning to be Old*, 36.

16. Carroll L. Estes et al., "The Medicalization and Commodification of Aging and the Privatization and

Rationalization of Old Age Policy," *Social Policy and Aging: A Critical Perspective*, ed. Carroll Estes and Associates (Thousand Oaks: Sage Publications, 2001): 46.

17. Carroll Estes, Charlene Harrington and David N. Pellow, "The Medical-Industrial Complex and the Aging Enterprise," Ch 8. *Social Policy and Aging* Thousand Oaks. Sage. 2007. 165 passim.

18. CTV News, "Hurried Women Syndrome a Real Problem, Says Doc," <http://www.ctv.ca/servlet/ArticleNews/Story/CTVNews/1040054302836 _52?/hub=Health> (accessed November 11, 2004).

19. Daphne Branham, "Another Epidemic," *Vancouver Sun*, October 30, 2004.

20. Ray Moynihan and Alan Cassels, *Selling Sickness: How the World's Biggest Pharmaceutical Companies are Turning us All Into Patients* (Vancouver: Greystone Books, 2005).

21. Ibid., vii.

22. Ibid., xi.

23. Susan A. McDaniel, "Sentenced by a Metaphor: Living With Aging," *Recent Advances, Research Updates* 6, 3 (2005): 275-8.

24. Martha B. Holstein, "A Feminist Perspective on Anti-Aging Medicine," *Generations* (Winter 2001-2): 38, 39.

25. Ibid., 41.

26. Maxwell J. Mehlman et al., "Anti-Aging Medicine: Can Consumers Be Better Protected?" *Gerontologist* 44, 3 (2004): 304.

27. Neal King, and Toni Calasanti "Empowering the Old: Critical Gerontology and Anti-Aging in a Global Context," in Jan Baars, et al *Aging, Globalization and Inequality: The new Critical Gerontology*. Amityville, New York. Baywood Publishing Company, Inc. (2006): 143.

28. Helen Branswell, "Openness in Drug Regulatory Process 'Grossly Inadequate'," *Globe and Mail*, November 23, 2004.

29. Prestwood, K.M., Editorial, "The Search for Alternative Therapies for Menopausal Women: Estrogenic Effects of Herbs," *The Journal of Clinical Endocrinology and Metabolism*, 88, 9 (2003): 4075.

30. Joan C. Callahan, "Menopause: Taking the Cures or Curing the Takes?" in *Mother Time: Women, Aging and Ethics*, ed. Margaret Urban Walker (Lantham: Roman and Littlefield Publishers, 1999), 151-174.

31. Ibid., 154.

32. Susan Love and Karen Lindsey, *Hormone Book: Making Informed Choices About Menopause* (NY: Random House, 1998). Note: A revised edition was published in 2003.

33. Callahan, op.cit., 164.

34. Boston Women's Health Collective, *Our Bodies, Ourselves*, 685.

35 Suzanne Somers, *Ageless: The Naked Truth About Bioidentical Hormones* (NY: Crown Publishers, 2006).

36. Leah McLaren, "Crissy Snow--health guru?" *Globe and Mail*, November 11, 2006.

37. Gloria Wade-Gayles, "Who Says an Older Woman Can't/Shouldn't Dance?" in *Body Politics and the Fictional Double*, ed. Debra Walker King (Bloomington and Indianapolis: Indiana University Press, 2000), 2.

38. Peggy Downes et al., *The New Older Woman: A Dialog for the Coming Century* (Berkeley, CA: Celestial Arts, 1996).

39. Sharon McIrvin Abu-Laban and Susan A. McDaniel, "Beauty, Status and Aging," in *Feminist Issues: Race, Class and Sexuality*, 4th Ed., ed. Nancy Mandell (Canada: Pearson

Education Canada, 2005), 113.

40. Suzanne Slater, *The Lesbian Family Life Cycle* (New York: Free Press, 1995), 221.

41. Olive Skene Johnson, *The Sexual Rainbow: Exploring Sexual Diversity* (London: Fusion Press, 2003), 62.

42. Cruikshank, *Learning to be Old*, 121.

43. Gary Geyer, "Being Gay or Lesbian and Past 50," <http://www.50plusmag.com/50plusissues/120104gaylesbian/120104gaylesbian.html> (accessed December 17, 2004).

44. Tony Atherton, "'Sexlady' Likes to Work at Home," *Ottawa Citizen*, reprinted in Vancouver Sun, March 13, 2004.

45. "Still Doing It," *The Passionate Eye*, CBC. dir. Deirdre Fishel and Diana Holtzberg (Transit Films) <http://cbc.ca/passionateeye/feature-2711/03.html> (accessed December 20, 2005). See also <http://www.stilldoingit.com>.

46. *Statistics Canada, Women in Canada: A gender-based statistical report* (5th Ed., Ottawa: Ministry of Industry, Catalogue no.89-5-3-XPE): 53. 2006.

47. Ibid., 54.

8. Ibid., 57.

49. Statistics Canada, Op.Cit.54.

50. Neena Chappelle et al., *Aging in Contemporary Canada* (Toronto: Prentice Hall, 2003), 258.

51. Ibid., 276.

52. Arlene Bierman, Aging Well: What Every Woman Should Know," <http://www.womenshealthmatters.ca/facts/quick_show_d?cf?number=450> (accessed July 19, 2006).

53. Richard Levandowski, *The Anti-Aging Combo: Fitness, Flexibility* <http://xxx.zwire.com/site/news.cfm?newsid=17480444BRD+1091&PAG=461&dept.> (accessed November 18, 2006).

54. Andrew V. Wister, *Baby Boomer Health Dynamics: How Are We Aging?* (Toronto, Buffalo, London: University of Toronto Press, 2005).

55. Wister, *Baby Boomer Health Dynamics*: 19-20.

56. Ibid., 155-159 passim.
57. Ibid., 169-171.

58. Jenny Morris, *Encounters with Strangers* (London: Women's Press, 1996), 1 passim.

59. Op.Cit. Statistics Canada, *Women in Canada*, 54-55.

60. Susan Wendell, *The Rejected Body: Feminist Philosophical Reflections on Disability* (New York and London: Routledge, 1996), 11.

61. Ibid., 12.

62. Bonnie Sherr Klein, *Slow Dance: A Story of Love and Disability* (Toronto: Alfred A. Knopf Canada, 1997).

63. Jon F. Nussbaum et al., "Ageism and Ageist Language across the Life Span: Intimate Relationships and Non-Intimate Interactions," Journal of Social Issues 61, 2 (2005): 287-304.

64. Ibid., 297.

65. Ewa Szumacher, "Women in Academic Medicine: New Manifestations of Gender Imbalances," <http//aries.oise.utoronto.ca/highered/include/getdocs. p;hp?id=196&article=40&mode-pdf: 4>.

66. Kirsteen R. Burton and Ian K. Wong, "A force to contend

with: the gender gap closes in Canadian medical schools,"
CMAJ 170, 9 (2004): 1385-1386.

67. Information provided by The Faculty of Medicine at the
University of Ottawa, The Office of Equity, Diversity, and
Gender Issues, <http://www.medicine.Uottawa.ca/
genderequity/eng/index.html> (accessed July 8, 2008).

68. Margaret Munro, "Older Women at risk in ICU: study,"
Globe and Mail, Nov. 15, 2007: 9A.

69. "Canada Health Act: Overview," *Health Canada*,
<http://www.hc-sc.gc.ca/medicare/chaover.htm>
(accessed November 14, 2004).

70. Robert Steinbrook, "Private Health Care in Canada," *The
New England Journal of Medicine*, 354: 1661-1664,
<http://content.nejgm.org/cgi/content/full354/16/16
61 Retrieved 9/29/2006> (accessed April 20, 2006).

71. Ibid., 2-3.

72. Ibid., 2.

73. Chappelle et al., op.cit., 426.

74. Ibid., 427.

75. News Online, Canadian Broadcasting Corporation

(CBC), February 2, 2005.

76. *Homecare in Canada*, Roy Romanow, Discussion Paper, Commission on the Future of Health Care in Canada. See also an analysis of *Home Care in Canada* Policy Statement, Canadian Association on Gerontology <http://www.cagacg.ca/publications/552_e.php> (accessed December 12, 2006).

77. Andre Picard, "Private ER issue still festers," *Globe and Mail*, December 7, 2006.

78. Michael Mendelson and Pamela Divinsky, *Canada 2015: Globalization and the Future of Canada's Health Care*, Prepared for the Future of Global and Regional Integration Project, Institute of Intergovernmental Relations, Queen's University, Caledon Institute of Social Policy, 2002, 3.

79. David Cheal, ed., *Aging and Demographic Change in a Canadian Context* (Toronto: University of Toronto Press, 2002), 5.

80. Harriet Jackson and Alison McDermott, "Healthcare Spending: Prospect and Retrospect, Analytical Note," (Ottawa, ON: Economic and Fiscal Policy Branch, Department of Finance, January 2004) <www.healthcoalition.ca/finance-note.pdf>.

81. Mendelson and Divinsky, *Canada 2015*, 35.

82. Statistics Canada, *Table Persons in low income before tax, by prevalence in percent*, <http:www40.statcan.ca/101.cst01/famil41a-eng.htm> (accessed May 6, 2008).

Chapter Four

Women, Work and Retirement: The work bone's connected to the wage bone . . .

"We may be eating catfood by candlelight!"
— A boomer woman's response
when asked about late life resources.

The term 'bag lady syndrome' is used to describe the dread some women have of not having enough money in retirement to maintain a reasonable standard of living, or worse of being destitute. Work and retirement are undoubtedly core concerns for mid-life baby boom women, and now that the leading edge of the boomer bulge has reached the age of sixty, the topic of retirement seems to permeate most other current boomer considerations. Opinions seem quite mixed: there are those who profess that baby boomers, given all the changes in recent decades, will have comfortable later lives, but others believe that a significant proportion will not sail into a golden sunset. Which position is closer to reality? The deciding factors will include women's paid work, their unpaid work, their family caregiving responsibilities, Canada's pension system, and its implications for their retirement. All of these are critically important for women's roadmaps.

Boomer women's lives are very different than that of their mothers, let alone their grandmothers. Women in those generations were socialized to stay by home and hearth and to fulfill themselves by nurturing other family members. Everyone else came first, and many of these women had to derive their satisfaction vicariously by helping others to achieve. This often came at great psychological cost, a fact that Betty Friedan demonstrated in her landmark book, *The Feminine Mystique*, which is credited with starting the women's movement of the 1960s and '70s. When these women did engage in paid work, it was usually either before marriage or after their children had grown, at which time they were categorized as "re-entry women" – a term probably unknown to boomer women. Men were proud of the fact that their wives didn't "have" to work, something that sounds comical today. As one of my focus group women put it succinctly, "We did what we were supposed to do" and the other group members nodded their heads in agreement.

But in the late 20th century, there was a surge of women into the paid labor force, a surge that occurred within the context of a major economic shift-globalization. It produced profound changes that affected both women and men, but more particularly women in relation to their involvement in both paid and unpaid work. What are some of the significant results of these changes?

The Work Bone's Connected to the Wage Bone

• Women now make up 46.8% of persons employed in Canada. The numbers of women over age fifteen in the ranks of employed women rose from 42% in 1976 to 54% in 1990.

• Of particular interest are the changes in age groups; in 2004 76% of women aged forty-five to fifty-four were employed, up from 46% in 1976.

• The share of women aged fifty-five to sixty-four – the older boomer cohort in the paid work force – rose from 30% to 46% between 1976 and 2004. Men's employment was higher than women's in both boomer age categories: forty-five to fifty four and fifty-five to sixty-four.

• In all age groups, women are more likely than males to work part-time. This is especially true of women between the ages of twenty-five to fifty-four. In 2004, 20% of both the twenty-five to forty-four and forty-five to fifty-four age ranges worked part-time, compared with less than 5% of men in each of the age groups. At the same time, in 2004 women aged fifty-five to sixty-four – the older midlife boomer cohort – were about three times as likely as men in the same age range – 30% versus 11% – to work part-time.

• There has been a particularly sharp growth in the employment rate of women with children in the past two decades. In 2004, 73% of all women with children under age sixteen living at home were part of the employed work force, up from 39% in 1976. This is a truly remarkable shift. In addition, there has been an increase in employment of women with very young children. In 2004, 65% of all women with children under three years were employed, more than double that of 1976, when only 28% were employed, and the vast majority of employed women with children held full-time jobs.

• Women have increased their representation in many professional fields. In 2004, 55% of all doctors and dentists in Canada were female, up from 43% in 1987. They have also increased their representation in business and financial professions, social sciences, and religious occupations, as well as managerial positions. However, among managers, women tend to be better represented in lower level as opposed to senior level positions.

• More women are self-employed. In 2002, 11% of all those with jobs were self-employed.

• Higher educational achievement increases the likelihood of women being employed. In 2002, 75% of those with a university degree and 69% of those with a certificate or diploma were employed compared to 60% of those with some post-secondary training and 60% of high school graduates.

• There has been a dramatic increase in dual-earner couples, accompanied by a gain in the number of wives who are primary breadwinners. In 1967, an estimated 11% of wives earned more than their husbands. By 2003 this proportion had nearly tripled to 29%. But wives who were primary breadwinners earned $41,200 in 2003, well below the level of $57,800 among their male counterparts. In general, primary earner wives earned less than primary earner husbands in each occupational group.

• In 2002-2003, 54% of children aged six months to five years were in some form of childcare, up from 42% in 1994-1995. Three forms of care – daycare centers, care outside the home by a non-relative and care by a relative either inside or outside the home – each accounted for around 30% of all children in child care.[1]

The scope of the changes embodied by these statistics is truly remarkable, and although like the old saw about not seeing the forest for the trees, they are all things that affect people in their daily lives. What is particularly encouraging is that these changes, which are of historic proportions, took place in a matter of twenty-eight years. And that fact is encouraging because it suggests that changes still needed may come about in a reasonably short period of time. Of particular significance for mid-life women is the number of increases in paid work by women aged forty-five to fifty-four and those fifty-five to sixty-four, representing earlier and later boomer women cohorts. Equally significant – in fact, jaw-dropping – are the number of women with small children who are in paid work. Also noteworthy are the number of children six months to five years who are cared for by a relative, whose availability can be less than reliable, given illness or availability of the caregiver. The percentage of part-time women workers has remained fairly steady since the 1970s, likely an indication of women's continued family responsibilities. Women may work part-time either by design (when it is the only type of work they want) or by default (when it is necessary because of family responsibilities, inability to find full-time work, or health problems).

It is no surprise that, on the whole, women earn less than men – some 71% of what men earn for full-time, full-year work. According to Statistics Canada, the difference between the percentage of their earnings, compared to that of men's has been fairly consistent from 1991 through to 2003. In 1991, it was 69.7% and in 2003, it was 70.5%.[2] Of course, earnings vary with age, educational attainment, skills and experience. Education pays big time, earnings are commensurate with education, and women with university degrees earn more. The Canadian economist Monica Townson notes that, if the wage gap for all earners, rather for just full-time, full-year earners, is considered, then women's average earnings are only 64% of those of their male counterparts.[3]

With the increase in "non-standard work" resulting from downsizing, restructuring, and outsourcing, the service sector has grown, and with it casual, contingent, contractual work and holding more than one such job. Women are over-represented in these "McJobs": in 2003, women held 40.4% of non-standard employment contrasted to men's 29.8%.[4] Such jobs are described as "precarious," which is no doubt an understatement.

Two issues that relate to possible future economic developments on mid-life boomer women's roadmaps are closely aligned: older workers and the expected shortage of workers. Over 300,000 Canadians aged sixty-five and over were employed in 2001, with older men outnumbering older women, 68% were men, and 57% were women. In 2001, one in twelve seniors had a job, and over four of ten employed were seventy or older. The lower rates for older women may reflect their lower education. The division of labor remains traditional, with women in these pension-aged categories working as secretaries and as child-minders. Still, as the researcher Doreen Duschene found, "despite living in an increasingly technological society, the more highly educated baby boomers can expect to qualify for more occupations than ever before as they approach retirement age."[5] This is an important observation for mid-life boomer women who may decide to work in later life, given that the work they do now requires technological sophistication, which will mean a wider range of occupations open to them later on. Reviewing a 2007 world wide report "HSBC Global Survey Reveals Billions contributed by Older People" Virginia Galt, May 23, 2007 in the *Globe and Mail* commented that half of those in their 40's and 50's planned to continue working as long as possible. This study of twenty-two countries included Canadian respondents aged forty to seventy-nine.

Given population aging, the aging of the workforce, and the forthcoming retirement of boomers, the topic of future labor shortages seems to be preoccupying policy makers, labor leaders, and the media. For example, a typical headline reads, "Retired Seniors viewed as Future Source of Labor to Fill Job Vacancies."[6] Another media source raised the spectre of huge disruptions to the national economy caused by a shortage of labor.[7] Both of these considerations, an aging labor force and possible shortages, could mean greater possibilities for women who choose to or need to continue working as they age. Work may become as central to women's lives as it has been for men. Apart from needed income, the self-worth, satisfaction, and self-esteem of work provides more than a measure of fulfillment. Education, training and experience are strong motivators for women who want to keep working. When I conducted some pre-retirement workshops on this topic a few years ago, one of the women said, "I have to keep working. If I stay at home now, I'll be wearing the same nightgown on Friday as I did on Monday morning." This intense declaration expresses how validated this woman is by her work and hence, her fear of stopping. Commenting on needed technological skills, one Statistics Canada report states, "It is probable that within the population as a whole, gender differences in work behavior are now substantially less important than the differences in skill levels."[8] This is good news for mid-life working boomers and their future work.

Flashpoints

Divorce, separation, or widowhood and finding themselves at the head of a single, female-headed family are some of the situations midlife women may face that could make them more vulnerable.

Divorce

In addition to the possible loss of social status, there is often a decline in financial resources – disproportionately so for women – upon being divorced. In a report for the Vanier Institute of the Family, Anne-Marie Ambert found that divorce is a direct cause of poverty for women and children. Canadian women's household incomes plummet by about 50% upon divorce, while men's decline by only 25%. Adjusted for family size, however, women's income drops by 40% while men's income increases slightly. Ambert also found that, even three years after divorce, women's incomes remain far below what they were during marriage.[9] It is not only the economic aspects, there is also the social stigma. I talked to a divorced boomer woman in her late fifties who had been married to a prominent physician, who then left her for a younger woman. She said "At first I wouldn't go out, and when I had to go shopping, I tied a kerchief around my head and put on dark sunglasses."

Interestingly, it appears that the high rate of divorce in Canada may be slowing somewhat. The number of divorces is now 11.2%, below what it was in 1992, though it is too early to tell whether this trend will continue.[10]

Further, divorces are occurring at later stages of life. In the U.S., some couples are even divorcing when in their eighties.

Canada seems to be following suit, according to an article in the *National Post*, "Sixty and Starting Over: Rise in Grey Divorce as Boomers call it quits." It notes that whereas the idea of ending a marriage after several decades may have been unthinkable for previous generations, "But Baby Boomers, particularly women in their 50's and 60's are advancing a new social trend – the grey divorce."

According to Barbara Mitchell, a Simon Fraser University professor who comments "that the overall divorce rate declined about 11% between 1993 and 2003. However it increased by 34% for those aged 50-54, about 50% for those aged 55-59, by about 30% for those aged 60-64, and about 9% for those aged 65 and older."[11] It seems like many women in late life don't want to tolerate unhappy marriages, and are chipping away at a perceived barrier to their independence on their roadmaps.

Widowhood

The death of a spouse is undoubtedly one of the most devastating events one can experience. Apart from the awful wrench, the decline in income and standard of living is onerous, particularly for senior women. In an analysis for Statistics Canada, Andre Bernard and Chris Li found that not only did widows' adjusted income decline, more of them fell below the low-income threshold following widowhood.[12] Their study, which compares the decline in income among senior women who remained married to the decline in income of widowed women, found that five years down the road, median family income had declined 9.8% among widowed women – a figure that is more than six times greater than the 1.5% decline among senior women who remained married. Once widows' incomes fall below the low-income threshold, it is hard for them to climb out. Not surprisingly, older widowers remarry more often than do older widows – widowers limited ability to look after themselves undoubtedly being a factor. However, given better health and the decreasing age gap in life expectancy between men and women, and given higher employment among mid-life women, these numbers may decrease.

Single parenthood

Single parent mothers account for the majority of all single parent families in Canada. Though the poverty rate has, thankfully, declined, the poverty rate for these single-parent mothers in 2003 was still 48.9%. The poverty rate for single-parent fathers is usually less than half the rate for female single-parent families.[13] In 2006, though incomes rose for female lone-parent families, still 42.6% (before tax) were considered to have low incomes.

The ways in which women become single-parent mothers are noteworthy. While in earlier years, it was the commonly held attitude that young sole mothers were in these difficulties because of their irresponsibility and penchant for wanting handouts, today it is clear that marriage breakdown is the main reason for the high rate of poverty among families headed by single-parent mothers. As with other issues, education and training in relation to getting jobs play a large part in these single mothers' financial circumstances. The gendered social structure, the financial consequences of divorce and separation and the lack of affordable childcare also play large roles. And the lone-parent mother who goes on social assistance may suffer a triple whammy, as it were. If she gets a job, depending on the province she lives in, she will lose as much as one dollar of assistance for every dollar earned, or be allowed to keep up to $100 or $200 of her earnings per month. There may be other 'clawbacks' according to where she lives.[14]

In 2004, Jean Pelletier, chief executive officer of Via Rail in Canada, made the following remarks about Miryam Bedard, a Canadian Olympic gold medallist: "I don't want to be mean but she is a poor girl who deserves pity, a girl who doesn't have a husband that I know of. She has the stress of being a single mother who has economic responsibilities. Basically I find that she deserves pity."[15] At the time Pelletier lost his job over this (he was later awarded damages for his dismissal), though probably only because the federal government was then mired in scandal and didn't need further cause for embarrassment; but whatever motivated his firing, his statement was appalling. It is not pity these women need, it is a revamping of our gendered social structure – a revamping that addresses the financial consequences for women of divorce, separation, and the lack of good affordable daycare. A few short years ago the popular US talk show host, Oprah Winfrey, had a number of single-parent mothers as guests, two of whom had lost their children in fires. The children had been left alone while their mothers worked the night shift so that they could stay at home and look after them during the day. In effect, these women lost their children because they feared losing their jobs. This is an extremely tragic story and thankfully is not typical, but it does tell us something about the invisible struggles of day-to-day experience for many single parent mothers. I know about this from my own experience, having lost my husband suddenly when he was forty-one years old, leaving me with two children, aged six and nine. I got a full-time job, which entailed a one-hour commute in each direction. I know what it feels like when you are rushing around at the breakfast hour and a child calls out in a thick voice, "Mummy, my throat hurts."

An interesting perspective comes from a report out of the Faculty of Social Sciences at McMaster University that found, with regard to poverty among unattached women, those who remain single fare better than do the widowed, the divorced or separated. In fact, among older unattached women in Canada, of those who are separated (including common-law relationships), widowed, divorced and single, those separated or divorced are the poorest. What is more, the burden of a low income in later years is heaviest on these unattached older women.[16] Lynn McDonald, an expert on women and aging who headed the study, in an interview with the *Vancouver Sun* spoke about the so-called "bag-lady syndrome" – the fear held by many women that old age will find them poverty stricken and on the street. She found that this fear is no joking matter, especially for elderly separated and divorced women. Widows faired lightly better than did divorced or separated women because some received spousal benefits and a share of assets.[17]

The Wage Bone's Connected to the Caregiving Bone . . .

A major part of the equation regarding women's paid work is their unpaid work, which is likely as important in the social and economic construction of women's late life resources as is their paid work. Much of this unpaid work is caregiving, a topic that has been widely written and talked about in popular, policy, and academic circles, yet somehow its economic effects are curiously downplayed. One analyst, writing in the *Journal of Comparative Studies*, has commented that "because it takes place in the privacy of households, is unpaid and is done by women, this critical activity is devalued and often unnoticed."[18] And Catherine Ward-Griffin and Victor Marshall note that caregiving is profoundly gendered. They express concern that, given cutbacks and a decline in formal care, a transfer of services will mean more care will fall on the family.[19] The family, of course, mainly means women, And this in turn means that mid-life baby boom women are right in the forefront, especially in the context of their own aging.

With the changing dynamics of families and steadily rising life expectancy comes the increased layering of generations occupying the same time space. Anne Martin-Matthews, a prominent Canadian scholar, puts it well when she says that "the period we know as old age for those who live to age 85 constitutes one quarter of their lives, and for those who live to age 95, one third of their lives! These are staggering proportions."[20] And it is women who form the majority of those living to be over 85. Thus, there are anecdotal scenarios wherein older women are looking after still older women, a 65-year-old, for example, caring for an 85-year-old parent in a wheelchair.

"Eldercare" is a term that many, including myself, do not like, because it seems to be parallel to child care, thus inferring need and dependency; however, it is a term now widely used. But for many boomer women, the reality is "double caregiving" because they are in the "sandwich generation," not only looking after children but also older family members. When we consider that there can now be four or five generations living in the same time space, there must be many women in this country looking after children, parents and grandparents. In my own and I'm sure many other older women's experience, being connected to a parent in her nineties as well as to adult children and grandchildren suggests that the term "clubhouse sandwich generation" would be more appropriate.

Looking at women's unpaid work in the global economic context, the highly respected Canadian sociologist Susan McDaniel points out that there is a "contradiction between the gendered dismantling of the welfare state and women's dramatic increase in paid work at the same time as more unpaid work is expected."[21] This, of course, is part and parcel of globalization and the shrinking of social support networks, which pull midlife caregivers in two directions. Some conservative policy makers and others with right-wing agendas, who suggest that a woman's "natural" role is as the caregiver within "the family," support the current neo-liberal emphasis on individual responsibility rather than collective approaches. The late, internationally renowned economist John Kenneth Galbraith – a Canadian by birth – used the term "convenient social virtue" to refer to the fact that the economic value of women's unpaid work is conveniently overlooked, the excuse being that, for women, virtue should be its own reward . This, as Galbraith suggested, is not the kind of reward that will ensure women's financial security in their later lives. It is also very "convenient" for those who support the regressive idea that women are born to be nurturers.

The question of the economic value of women's unpaid work is raised from time to time by some social analysts, but never seems to become a focal point of serious attention. This is how Malika Hamdad has calculated it for Statistics Canada: the estimated value of unpaid household work in Canada in 1998 was $297 billion. Of all unpaid work 94% occurred inside the household, the remaining 6% outside the household. The value per person of unpaid housework was estimated to be $12 256, which comes to $15 101 dollars per woman versus $9319 per man. She also compared the gender differences between those who were employed and those who were not. Women who were not employed contributed the greatest proportion of the value of unpaid household work: 36%. Those who were employed contributed 27%. Employed men contributed 22%, while unemployed men contributed 15%.[22]

Another aspect was presented in a Canadian report by Katherine Marshall in 2006. She found that gender roles were converging, with men now taking on more of the unpaid work. The proportion of those doing some housework daily increased from 72% in 1986 to 79% in 2005; the now more common dual-earning families could account for this rise in men's participation, certainly a move in the right direction. Women, however, still shoulder the bulk of the work at home.[23] A rather tongue-in-cheek 2006 US estimation of the value of women's unpaid work, entitled "What is Your Mom Worth?" or the "Mom job" as the writer calls it, estimated that stay-at-home moms should earn $134 121 annually, while working moms should earn $85 876 annually for the "mom job" portion of their work, in addition to their actual "work job."[24]

So what does this unpaid work entail, and how can it be valued? Here is a scenario: Vivian is in her early forties and works full-time as a supervisor in the education department of the city's central school system. She and her partner can both take a large number of days off as part of parental leave, which is partially paid and which can be used to look after a sick child. They have two children, aged nine and twelve. At seven am, Vivian is getting dressed and preparing breakfast one day when one of the children throws up and announces she feels hot. Vivian is making an important presentation that day, and since her husband is out of town, she decides against using her parental leave days and calls the local daycare agency, which is part of the public education system, to arrange for someone to come over. She also utilizes a nearby help agency to come later in the day, shop, and prepare dinner.

A fantasy about family life on the Planet Zog? Well, yes and no. In fact, a number of such basic service structures are in place on *this* planet, though largely in Nordic countries. For example, Sweden provides paid leave for parents of up to forty-eight days shared equally between partners, and up to sixty days for a parent who has to take time off work to attend to a sick or special needs child. There is also temporary parental benefit if the person who looks after the child is ill.[25] Of course, the little scenario above is a fantasy and an exaggeration, and things would probably not go quite so smoothly, but the point is that forms of it do exist elsewhere, in countries that recognize the value of unpaid work and have social policies to support those values. Canada does have parental leave availability under its Employment Insurance provisions. Mothers are the main users, but some fathers, approximately 10% of the total are increasingly utilizing these benefits. It was amusing to hear from a 30-year-old new father, the son of an older couple I know, who took leave to look after his six-month-old daughter when his wife went back to her job. He observed that "if men had always to do all the housework, there would be national day care in short order." This may contain more truth than appears on the surface.

Given longevity and changes to family structures, the issue of needful older parents and other relatives looms large for mid-life boomers' roadmaps. With regard to changes in family dynamics, as Ward-Griffin and Marshall suggest, care provision for the elderly, requires new conceptualization."[26] Indeed it does. One of the impacts of caregiving for Canadian seniors with long-term health problems is the move away from institutional care: fewer than 10% of senior women and fewer than 5% of senior men are in institutions. Most live in the community, leaving the bulk of caregiving duties to family and friends. One in five Canadians forty-five years and over provide informal care to a senior.[27] Keeping in mind the rise in the number of women aged forty-five to sixty-four now in the paid workforce, the implications suggest a time crunch for boomer women, now and to come.

Canada does not have a national home care program, though this issue is widely discussed. As a result, home care differs across the provinces and is a mix of public, private, for- profit and not-for profit services and family providers (for Compassionate Care, see Appendix 1). In fact, according to data released on the 2006 Census, Statistics Canada found that there has been an increase in the numbers of Canadians doing some form of unpaid senior care in 2006, with 18.6 per cent of Canadians doing so, contrasted to 16.5% in 1996. These numbers will undoubtedly continue to rise.

In fact, a 2008 Canadian study provides details in a first time study which corroborates this dynamic.[28] Analyzing data from 2007, it found that 43% were men and 57% were women. A further 57% were working at a paid job.[29] This study offers rich details on who are involved, family members, the types of infirmity the care receivers have, seniors caregiving other seniors, tasks undertaken and more.

There is, of course, far, far more to looking after older parents than the percentages and activities shown above that make it all appear somewhat mechanistic. The majority of adult children who provide care to their parents do so with devotion and concern, whether that care is informal or formal. "I wouldn't have it any other way," is the comment that sums up the feelings of most of the caregivers in my focus groups. These women had strong feelings around "giving something back," an indication of both intergenerational reciprocity and deep affection.

The positive aspects of caregiving – such as increased closeness, deepening of bonds and greater understanding – need to be recognized. In fact, one of the most gut-churning life experience for many is having to place a parent in an institution.

Caregiving tasks are significantly gendered, with men more likely to perform the tasks outside the home – for example, house repairs, yard work, and painting – while two thirds of personal caregiving – or "intense care" – is performed by females. The latter includes such time-consuming tasks such as bathing, toileting, and cutting nails. At the same time, the caregiver will generally be carrying out a full agenda of household work. Frida Furman provides a glimpse of what is involved in this: meal planning and preparation, grocery shopping , vacuuming, dusting, scrubbing, wiping, dish washing, toilet cleaning, bed making, floor washing and waxing, laundry, folding and ironing, window washing, general pick-up and straightening, garbage disposal, minor repairs, paying bills, purchasing miscellaneous products.[30] (Just typing this list is tiring.)

"I've cooked fifteen turkeys by telephone." This comment, made by a boomer woman I talked to, typifies the feelings of those who juggle paid and unpaid work. A former co-worker of mine who is in her fifties, single and working full-time as a secretary, tends her mother who lives with her and is in the early stages of dementia. She does get a few hours a day of homecare. I asked her, "Do you ever get out to a movie, or concert or go shopping?" She replied, "No, I can't afford it. I'd have to find a compatible caregiver who wouldn't upset mother, at a cost of about fifteen dollars per hour. It just isn't worth it."

Another example comes from a woman in her early sixties who attends to her Alzheimer's-stricken husband but continues to do consulting from her home. In order to attend a two-day conference that was important for upgrading in her field of work, she had to pay $450 for a suitable caregiver for her husband, this being in addition to the costs of the conference. Another mid-life boomer woman in the paid workforce uses what she calls "Pot Roast Therapy" when her housekeeping time suffers due to other responsibilities. This dish is obviously a family dinner favourite that she offers as consolation for what she considers her neglect of them. It would more appropriate, however, if some other family member put some energy into both alleviating such feelings of guilt and preparing a nice dinner for her after a hard day.

A report by Wendy Pyper on people who juggle both paid and unpaid work was aptly titled "Balancing career and care."[31] Pyper examined caregiving to seniors and found that 1.7 million Canadian adults aged forty-five to sixty-four provided informal care in 2002 to almost 2.3 million older relatives and noted that 70% of these caregivers (both men and women) were also employed. And since life expectancy is still increasing, she feels that many of these mid-life caregivers will not only continue working but will also continue to act as caregivers for extended periods. At the same time, combining a heavy workload, family support and day-to-day tasks may lead to fatigue or to quitting a job earlier than expected.[32] She uses the term "high intensity" caregiving to mean those who spend four hours per week at it, based on a forty-hour work week, and notes that such caring can lead to changes in social activities, holiday plans, or sleep patterns, in addition to incurring extra expenses. When respondents were asked if caregiving had caused them to reduce the hours they worked, change their work patterns, or turn down a job offer or promotion, 37% of the women and 24% of the men said yes. These people also suffered feelings of guilt for not doing more, and a huge proportion – 82% – reported sometimes or nearly always feeling stressed while balancing their responsibilities. Finally, and certainly very seriously for mid-life caregivers, 21% of women aged 45-64 and

11% of similarly aged men who were not yet retired stated that caregiving was one of the reasons for their upcoming retirement. Among those already retired in the same age group, 21% of the women and 8% of the men acknowledged that providing needed care to a family member was among their reasons for retiring. Overall, Pyper found that 70% of these caregivers stated their life satisfaction level was good or excellent, though this appeared to me to be somewhat of a contradiction, given the high level of guilt and stress reported. Perhaps these caregivers and many others are not comfortable complaining as it is their parents and other older relatives who are the recipients. Whatever the reasons for their conflicted feelings, it is clear that these midlife caregivers pay a significant price both in economic and psychological terms. The eldercare study cited above notes some of the strains which add to their stress.

John Kenneth Galbraith's criticism of unpaid work as a "convenient social virtue" looms large in this context. It is convenient in that the work gets done and convenient economically in that it also gets ignored. A tongue-in-cheek, lighthearted reflection about the value of "Mom's" household work," or "What is Mom Worth?" mentioned above, diverts one from the serious significance of the underlying social and economic structures and it's possible large costs to many midlife caregivers. Given unpaid caring, population aging, lack of affordable daycare and inadequate home care arrangements, mid-life boomer women – and to growing extent men – are being pulled in two directions. And this will likely continue. Paramount to mid-life women's roadmap is that they are called upon and will continue to perform unpaid caregiving exactly *at the same time as they need to be saving and otherwise getting ready for their own retirement.* It is to this difficulty that I now turn.

The Caregiving Bone's Connected to the Pension Bone . . .

Canada has a strong pension system, which is admired as a model of a successful mix of public and private pensions. But I have heard numerous women say they find the pension system confusing and difficult to sort out. And with good reason, since the terminology is obscure except to those who are familiar with it, such as certified general accountants and actuaries. This leaves most people out.

So how does one begin to sort out the OAS, the GIS, the CPP, the Allowance, RRSPs, group RRSPs , RPPs and all the rest of the alphabet soup of pension and retirement benefits?

First, it will be necessary to make reference to the many changes to the pensions systems which have been and are being made globally. Such pension reforms reflect the public's concern about aging populations and the ability to pay benefits when the boomer bulge retires. And now that the leading edge boomers have turned sixty, we hardly see a daily newspaper without some reference to pensions and retirement; in fact, it has become a media preoccupation.

Boomer women are understandably concerned given their huge numbers in the paid work force and their impending retirement sometime before the year 2031. There is much, therefore, to gain from focusing on the system itself in terms of what can be expected, what improvements would be helpful and what roles women can play towards their later life security. Think of the following then as bad-tasting cough syrup, hard to take in, but helpful.

Among pension reforms occurring in many countries are two that stand out because of their far-reaching consequences.

The first is the move from defined benefits to defined contributions. In a defined benefit system the amount of pension benefits a person will receive on retirement can be clearly calculated, based on previous work history and contributions she/he has made. The ability to know what one can expect is crucial to planning one's late-life resources. In a defined contributions system, one's pension contributions are market-based; this means that the final benefits cannot be known in advance because they are based on market values, which are, to say the least, fluid. Think Nortel and Enron, and now the devastating 2008 financial meltdown.

A second major global reform involves the move towards privatization of public pension funds, meaning that a part of each person's contributions would be invested in "individual accounts" and once again open to market vagaries.

The United States has been considering – on and off – privatizing aspects of its Social Security system, but the idea has not met with much public support. Basically, privatization involves moving away from public pensions in order to place more financial responsibility on individuals.

Older women and men, especially those with insufficient means who are already close to the poverty line, would be most vulnerable. An American umbrella group of women's advocates, which includes many who are familiar with the law as it relates to social security, cautions that privatization would see a decrease in traditional benefits – "an event that could spell disaster, particularly for elderly women who live alone and 25% of whom rely on Social Security as their sole income."[33]

In Canada, privatization of pensions would negatively affect the over 37% of unattached women sixty-five and over who live at or close to the poverty line as well as the single parents and families not covered by occupational pensions.

To date Canada has not made such moves, although there are those who are red-flagging this possibility. The Canada Pension Plan (CPP) made changes in 1997 by raising contributions to cover the expected number of boomer retirements, a move that should relieve the it-won't-be-there-when-I-need-it anxiety that many boomers are experiencing. A second change was the establishment of a CPP Investment Board, at arms length from the government, that is charged with investing CPP funds "prudently and responsibly" to insure its viability. According to Donald Raymond "This investment challenge will grow with the size of the CPP fund, estimated by the chief actuary of Canada to increase to $250 billion in 2016."[34]

Canada's pension system is commonly described as having three tiers or pillars, or is said to be "a three-legged stool."

The first tier includes Old Age Security (OAS) which pays a monthly income to all Canadians over sixty-five who meet the requirements. The Guaranteed Income Supplement (GIS) is a supplement paid to low-income pensioners or those with no other source of income, and the Allowance (AL) for those aged sixty to sixty-four for spouses or common-law partners of OAS pensioners. It should be noted that both the GIS and the Allowance are means-tested but not taxed. The costs of this first tier come out of the general tax base.

The second tier of the Canadian pension system is the retirement pension, called the Canada and Quebec Pension Plans (C/QPP – hereafter referred to as the CPP). Contributions are mandatory for all paid workers over the age of eighteen and are made by both the employer and the employee; the current rate is 9.9%, divided between the two (or 4.5% each). These contributions are tax deductible. Benefits are based on earnings and the length of time in the paid workforce. CPP benefits are based on a formula with a ceiling of 25% of the average wage, or maximum pensionable earnings which in 2008 was $44 900.[35] Many believe erroneously that the CPP is also funded from the tax base, but it is important to note that the CPP does not come from the general tax base but is funded by contributions from workers and their employers, from the self-employed and from investment earnings of the CPP's Investment Board – a crucial distinction from the funding of the OAS et al. The CPP is considered to be "woman friendly" because in addition to retirement benefits, it also provides death benefits, survivor's benefits, benefits for children and disability benefits.

The third tier of the pension system consists of the Registered Retirement Savings Plan (RRSP), the Registered Pension Plan (RPP) (which is also referred to as a workplace pension), the group RRSP, and the Registered Retirement Investment Fund (RRIF). All of the third tier plans are registered with the Canada

Customs and Revenue Agency for tax purposes, as well as with the federal and provincial pension authorities. (For more details please see Appendix 2.)

What's Wrong With This Picture? A Critique

The epigraph at the beginning of this chapter was the semi-serious answer given to me by a fifty-something employed boomer woman when I interviewed her about her late-life security. It displays a level of uncertainty about her – and in this case her partner's – abilities to meet their needs in later life. A closer look at the pension system is required to see how valid this apprehension is, and its relation to caregiving.

Of all eligible older Canadians 95% receive the OAS, which in 2008 averaged $476.36 per month. Women are more likely than men to receive the GIS, which in 2008 varied in amount according to eligibility: a single person received $437.37 and the spouse of an Allowance recipient averaged $355.95.[36] The OAS has an income ceiling when any person who receives $64 718 in income, in 2008, gets "clawed back," meaning she or he has to give back a portion of their OAS. If the income is $104 903 then the entire OAS pension is eliminated. I have often wondered why approximately $65 000 is considered to be wealthy if one is a senior, when in general, an income in the $85 000s is currently taken to be more in the order of wealth, but according to some even that is considered a conservative estimate. Currently, then, older women rely heavily on government transfers for their incomes. We can expect that when the majority of boomer women retire, having been in the workforce for longer periods, this reliance on government transfers may be far less.

Before looking at the second tier, the CPP, a glance at third tier RPPs or workplace pensions is helpful. Happily, more women in the paid work force are now covered by RPPs than was formerly the case. Whereas men previously accounted for almost 58% of the paid workforce, by the end of 2002 that number had declined to 53.6%, while the number of women in it had increased to 46.8%. This may reflect job losses for men, possibly following the current penchant for "outsourcing" and restructuring and the increase in the casual workforce. According to Statistics Canada, after only a modest gain in 2005 registered pension plans resumed normal growth in 2006 entirely the result in the increases among women.[37] In 2006, 38.9% of women paid workers, and 37.5% of men were covered by a registered pension plan (RPP).[38]

The downside is that close to 60% of women in the paid workforce are *not covered* by workplace pensions. One likely reason is that many work for small firms in the service sector. In fact, economist Monica Townson estimated that less than 20% of workers in the service sector were covered by employer-sponsored pension plans.[39] It is important to know if one is actually in a workplace pension plan, and employers, human resource departments or unions can readily provide this information. A few years ago a colleague and I wrote a short booklet containing the kind of information widows should have with regard to their finances – wills, pensions, and survivors benefits. One woman subsequently wrote to us to say that, based on the information in our booklet, she checked out her eligibility for a certain source of financial compensation we had mentioned and after due consultation received $6000 that she didn't know was owing to her. This is almost as good as winning the 6/49 lottery. Getting information, though often a tedious procedure, is a basic requirement for baby boom women's roadmaps.

RRSPs are a popular means of acquiring retirement savings, and women are increasingly turning to them. In 2005 men's median contribution was $3200, while women contributed $2300.[40] In 2007, men's median contribution was $3260 and women's $2300 virtually unchanged (these amounts were calculated before the Wall Street financial meltdown in 2008, when many savers and investors lost considerable sums).[41] One reason may be that RRSPs are open to all earners, unlike RPPs which are subject to availability, and obviously it is the high earners who contribute most. Thus, those who earn around $20 000, many of whom are women, are not heavy contributors. In fact, among lone mothers age thirty-five to fifty-four, those with top earnings contributed close to $5000 in 2003, while those at the lower end of the income scale contributed only $200. Wives who hold jobs with good pay and benefits have increasingly contributed to RPPs.[42] Those participating should keep in mind that RRSPs are a savings plan, not a pension, have no survivor's benefits, and are subject to the ups and downs of the market. Funds can be withdrawn when need arises, but this, of course, lessens the amount saved, and such takeouts are subject to tax. Although there are critics who feel the government should be getting the deferred taxes, given the near-hysteria on the part of financial institutions who flog RRSPs every February – including all the usual suspects: TV, radio, newspapers, magazines – if this clamour is any indication of their value to huge financial corporations, we can expect RRSPs to continue.

Turning now to the second tier, the CPP is compulsory, of growing importance to women in the paid workforce, and thus a major player in the Canadian pension system. It has been termed "woman friendly" because it has what is called the "seven-year drop out" provision, which allows a parent to take seven years off work to stay home and raise a child until she or he is seven years old. This means that the missed contributions during those non-working years are not counted. Other important aspects of the CPP include survivor's benefits, disability benefits, orphan's or child's benefits, and a death benefit. It is also portable, which means that it goes with the contributor when she/he changes jobs anywhere within Canada. It also allows for the splitting of pension benefits upon divorce or retirement.

Canada's pension system has been very successful in lowering poverty among seniors. By 2001 poverty rates had dropped – in fact, plummeted – from 39% to 16.8% of the population, that of unattached senior women went from over 70% to just over 45%, while that of unattached senior men fell from 61% to close to 33%.[43] However, any lessening of benefits would have serious consequences, especially since older single women are still among Canada's poorest. The importance of the system, though far from ideal, cannot be stressed too much, and to be blunt, it means that mid-life women and men need to keep current with any proposed changes. For example, detractors argue that, since so many women are now in the paid workforce, they are likely well-covered by pensions; the implicit suggestion being that perhaps part of the system is no longer needed. Of course, this is simply wrong-headed as almost 60% of women do not have employer pensions. In addition, Monica Townson suggests there are those who are now promoting the idea of increasing the age of retirement to sixty-seven as the US is doing, as well as advocating some privatization.[44] This is indeed a red-flag issue for boomer women, an issue that could understandably send them storming Parliament Hill. As this is unlikely at present, then keeping a wary eye on such proposals is a good beginning.

Given the number of women now in the labor force, what is the difference – or is there any – between what CPP benefits they get and what male workers get? The answer, unfortunately, is a resounding yes, there is a difference.

As of April, 2008 the monthly average retirement pension for men was $612.77, and that for women was $368.91. For the newly retired the amounts were $556.45 for men and $372.21 for women.[45]

However, according to a relevant study of newly retired women aged sixty-five to sixty-nine, the gap is closing.[46] This is encouraging, particularly for higher earning women, but given the persistent inequality of labor force earnings, the continuing large number of part-time workers and the unpaid work of female caregivers, the narrowing of the gap may proceed at glacial speed – or rather, now that glaciers are melting more quickly, it is probably more accurate to say that it may narrow with slug-like speed.

Pensions reflect the intertwining of a woman's age, marital status, occupations, earnings, and length of time in and out of the labor force for family responsibilities. On the surface, the system appears to be gender neutral, that is, it doesn't distinguish between men and women. In actuality this is not the case. As Lynn McDonald, an expert in women and aging, has found, "Policies simultaneously based on the worn-out breadwinner model, the cornerstone of 19th century industrial society and the gender neutrality of an earnings-related national pension system of the 20th Century ignore the gendered division of labor, which is at the heart of women's economic inequality in retirement."[47] In other words, though family and work have changed, women continue to be primary and unpaid caregivers, and such unpaid work will likely increase for mid-life women given aging parents and other relatives. For the CPP to be truly "woman friendly" and move towards the achievement of gender equality in pension benefits, unpaid caregiving and the ensuing loss of income must be recognized.

Finally, a word to relieve the anxiety created by the media-generated bombardment to the effect that the CPP will be unable to meet the needs of those retiring in the future due to aging workers and their pending retirement. Such is not the opinion of the Chief Executive officer of the CPP, John MacNaughton. He thinks that the CPP can be sustained for another seventy-five years: "There was a lot of talk about its viability and my sense is that the bad news got more publicity than the good news. We have every confidence that the plan is sustainable, but I guess that is less of a front-page story than if it were about to go over a cliff."[48] Despite continued assurance from CPP officers, the incorrect assumption "that it won't be there when I need it" persists, triggering unwarranted anxieties.

Mistruths die hard. Seventy-five years should take us to the year 2080, and the boomer retirement bulge ends in 2031. Sustainability of the pension system is also the opinion of a number of other experts. They suggest that those who promulgate fears about population aging fail to stress a number of important positive points: retired persons pay taxes, as they also do when RRSPs are withdrawn (some $4 billion in 2002) also on RIFFs; they no longer use the education system or unemployment insurance, and given the accumulated wealth now in pension systems, what boomers will require in pension benefits should balance what current workers contribute. Other than a national calamity, this balance should continue.

The Pension Bone's Connected to the Retirement Bone . . .

Though this section overlaps with the previous one, it is necessary to make it separate chiefly because the question of retirement and factors contributing to it are shifting rapidly, rather in the manner of tectonic plates. These shifts combine with the changing nature of the work force, especially because of the large number of women employed and their varied circumstances.

In fact, a rather breezy newspaper headline in the *Vancouver Sun* introducing an article by Anne Marie Owens with the words, "Women Transforming way Canadians retire" may not be at all far-fetched.[49] What is now referred to as "The New Retirement" may indeed reflect midlife women's working and retirement needs, another important signpost on their roadmap.

Retirement is and has really always been gendered. In general, women have retired earlier than men. By the 1980s, men were retiring at earlier and earlier ages, assisted by a change in the CPP that allowed retirement at age sixty as well as by new retirement incentives.

Then, in 2003, the median age of retirement for both sexes reversed directions, rising significantly for men though less so for women, possibly related to a downward slide in the economy. In 2007 the median age of retirement was 61.4 for men and 60.6 for women."[50]

Many women and men can't wait to retire. They may be sick of the daily grind or be in poor health; they may want to have more and different experiences, spend more time with family and friends, or travel. Golf and tennis may beckon. Some may want to volunteer in the community, while others may want to become "pro bono professionals." One woman in my focus groups remarked that "they [retirees] can go bungee-jumping if they want to." In fact, a friend of mine did exactly that to celebrate his seventy-fifth birthday. For those whose lives have come together in positive ways, retirement can be the clichéd "golden years," but this may be out of reach for others.

The timing of retirement is an issue that has been widely studied. In past years women would frequently retire when their husbands did, but with so many couples now being dual career earners, other considerations will affect the retirement decision. And this becomes another way women are affecting retirement. With the increased importance of work in the lives of boomer women, retirement may be neither what they want or what they need. Single women make the decision to retire themselves, but lack of pension coverage and fewer savings for those widowed, divorced or separated will mean that many will likely need to continue earning.

To Retire or Not to Retire (and when), That is the Question

Freedom 55 was a term coined by a financial institution to indicate that, with proper planning, meaning by using that company's services, one could retire by age 55. This was one of the greatest marketing ploys ever. But a survey of over 1500 baby boomers that Jonathan Chevreau, a columnist for the *National Post*, examined, revealed that most didn't expect to retire until very much later than that.[51] And when this question was raised in my focus groups, it was greeted with hoots of laughter. "Freedom 85 is more like it!" was how one woman expressed her reaction.

The "Freedom 55" banner heralding early retirement is in contrast to current realities of mid-life boomers. A study in which I was involved in 2000 looked at two groups of women, the first already retired and the second pre-retirees. It showed that some women who had already retired did so because of caregiving responsibilities. However, the second group – the pre-retirees – had not considered this possibility when they thought about the timing of their retirement.[52] A later study by Statistics Canada in *The Daily*, September 9 2008, and reported in the *Globe and Mail* September 10 2008, found 27% of those aged fifty to fifty-four plan to retire between sixty and sixty-four, 25.4% plan to retire at sixty-five or older, and 22.4% either don't know, or don't intend to retire. Thus this later study indicated that the uncertainty about retirement is continuing. There was a strong co-relation among those who had consulted financial advisors and those who felt their retirement was more secure. However, one expert, Terence Yuen, stated they may be over-confident, by underestimating the amount of money they will actually need to cover their living costs in retirement.

These findings are hardly a surprise and they indicate important things. First, given so many uncertainties, such as how to predict the future health of aging parents or the needs of adult children, it is difficult for many pre-retirement women to make plans. Second, as has been shown, social structures and the persistent division of labor in both the home and the workforce penalize women through the mismatch between their work and the pensions they receive.

The End of Retirement?

With the changes in the nature of work and the growth of non-standard, casual employment, the idea of "a job for life" is rapidly disappearing.[53] In fact, it is estimated that boomers and those who follow may hold as many as six jobs in a working lifetime.

This huge change, which could be called an upheaval, correlates with life course changes. In the past there was a three-part lifecourse pattern: (1) a period of education (2) a long period of work, and then (3) retirement. Now it is more likely to be a longer period of education, followed by working at several jobs, and a retirement that, rather than a one-time, finite work exit, is more like a series of labor force ins and outs. There is a longer transition from employment to final retirement, with patterns variously referred to as "pathways to retirement," "the new retirement," and "transitions to retirement." Some describe the process as having "bridge jobs" or as "zig-zagging" to retirement.[54]

This emerging pattern of labor force ins and outs in a sense mimics women's traditional work patterns. As Lynn McDonald puts it, "the transformation in retirement that we are witnessing today is, at bottom, women's retirement. In the past women's retirement was amorphous and fluid and is likely to continue to be so in the future, but for different reasons."[55] Among those reasons are the positive ones that baby boom women are better educated, many have good earnings and pensions, and having been in the workforce most of their adult lives may be more attached to the work they are doing and the fulfillment it brings. Also, with the large number of women in the service sector working in precarious jobs, there is the expectation they may need to continue working. For some women, leaving work can be a transition to the unpaid job of caregiving. Given both these streams – those who want to keep on working, those who have to keep on working – we can expect women to effect different retirement patterns. In fact, the occurrence of bridging, transitional jobs and zigzagging in and out of the labor force makes retirement more of a process.

A number of those who have left work, either

voluntarily or involuntarily, may return to work, some full-time, some part-time, not only for the income but because they want to be occupied – which is another type of need. Townson finds that those who return to the workforce will very likely hold non-standard jobs, be self-employed, or take part time or temporary jobs.[56] While there is understandable concern about the jobs some older workers take and the poor pay they receive in places like Walmart, there are psychological benefits that should not be underestimated even though they are not paid adequately. Older women and men who are hired as "greeters," security guards, or sales clerks (with the perky title of "retail sales associate") receive some needed income and are able to do something productive and enjoy the camaraderie of co-workers. And both of these extras are very important for self-respect and feelings of independence.

Bismarck Meets the Boomers

In 1891, Chancellor Otto Von Bismarck drew up legislation for old-age pensions, which were to be available to German civil servants when they reached age sixty-five. It was a canny move, as in those days men seldom lived that long. In numerous countries, and now thankfully including Canada, the discriminatory practice of requiring people to retire at age sixty-five has been recognized for the anachronism that is, and has been abolished. Possible future labor shortages are undoubtedly one of the reasons for this. A city bus passed me very recently which had painted across the top and along the full length of the bus "Why not make work part of your retirement?" This is indeed ironic, given the ageism in regard to older workers, particularly women.

However, there is a recent finding from the Canadian census of 2006 that older workers (aged sixty to sixty-four) are staying in the work force longer. The study suggests "that the labor force participation among this age group will continue to rise because of three factors: a strong attachment to the labor market among baby boomers; rising levels of education, particularly among women; and an apparent desire among people over 55 to continue working, either from interest, financial concern, or other factors, such as the virtual elimination of mandatory retirement at age 65."[57] Another study corroborates this trend noting that baby boomers may not be collectively fleeing freedom 55. The study notes that those aged fifty-five to sixty-four represented 11 percent of older workers in 1976, but was 14% in 2006: a proportion expected to grow as the baby boom generation ages. Further, the authors noting gender differences, found that men's participation rates at age fifty-five to fity-nine were lower in 2006 than previously, while women of the same age saw their participation rates climb. It appears, then, that the arguments made in this chapter about the need or desire of boomers to keep on working are beginning to materialize. Of course, these findings will have to be pursued for future trends.

However, another possibility looms which is the consideration of increasing the age at which pension benefits are available. The CPP as noted can start (with benefit loss) at age sixty, and continue (with benefit gain) to age seventy. There is the possible consideration of raising the age at which retirement benefits can be received from the standard of sixty-five to sixty-seven. The United States is already in process of doing this. Many concerned with feminist issues raise the question of how such a move would affect women, for example, with regard to their OAS and GIS eligibility. Raising the age of retirement to sixty - seven would mean that low income women would have to keep working longer until they are eligible. For others, it might mean an opportunity to keep earning and continue to contribute to their pension plan if they have one, as well as to receive their current salaries. Boomer women for whom raising the age to sixty-seven will be a roadblock on their route to retirement, should be aware of this possibility.

We're Mad as Hell and Not Going to Take it Any More

How will all these issues play out with respect to midlife women, some of whom are quickly approaching retirement? What role, if any, will they play in moving towards equity in the division of labor both in the home and in the workforce? Here are some thoughts:

- It is crucial that policy makers fashion a method that gives caregivers some pensionable credit for their work. At present, many caregivers have to cut back their paid work hours, work part-time, give up promotions, or quit work altogether. All of these options culminate in lower retirement benefits.

- The CPP should incorporate an up to three-year dropout period for workers who need to look after frail parents or other family members. This would be similar to the current seven-year dropout (Child Rearing Provision) period available to parents who are looking after pre-school children, a period that does not result in lower pension benefits.

• The present amounts of the OAS and GIS should be increased to bring poorer women and men to a level higher than the poverty line.

• RIFF regulations requiring set withdrawals should be revised, to allow RIFF holders more control. Forcing RIFF participants to take out set amounts may be against their best financial interests, especially given increased longevity and market uncertainty.

Of course, even if a number of these changes do come into being, some of which have already been raised by women's advocates, they are really only Band-Aids. A study conducted by four prominent Canadian academics concludes: "Finally predictions about the future must always be treated cautiously, especially when we are focusing on cohorts that will not enter retirement for another ten to twenty years. Based on our analysis, however, we conclude that most of tomorrow's older women, like today's, will not be financially secure in later life unless they are married."[58]

Unfortunately, this is far from being theoretical according to a recent study reported by Frances Bula in the *Globe and Mail,* September 18th, 2008, in an article entitled "When Golden Girls lose it all" (also reported in the National Post with the heading "Women, baby boomers swell ranks of Vancouver's homeless, report finds"). The study found among those aged fifty-five and over an increasing number were homeless, with older women being especially vulnerable. Although many such women's lives have been dysfunctional, the report noted that older women are less likely to have pensions or saved money than men left on their own. The same holds true for other provinces.

This chapter is not intended to be an exercise in victimology – quite the reverse. Women are not hapless victims; they are not Stepford Wives. Quite the contrary. For generations they have adapted their lives as circumstances have required. Mid-life boomer women are now participating in the making of history but may not be aware of the momentous changes that are affecting them and that they, in turn, are affecting, As Lynn McDonald points out in her paper *Invisible Retirement*, "It seems likely that the baby boom women born between 1947 and 1966, whose labor force participation will span most of their adult life for the first time in history, will be the earliest cohort of women to retire on mass *and their history is quite likely in the making*" (emphasis added).[59] These are powerful words, indeed a wake-up call for boomer women as they traverse their roadmaps and who are also potentially powerful because of their large numbers: four and a half million. The difference in CPP pension benefits makes it clear that at present women are getting about three-fifths of what men get. This simply mirrors both the reality of gender differences in the workforce and a mismatch between women's work and pension benefits.

In a recent book about women's retirement, *Women Confronting Retirement*, two of the writers, Nancy Dailey and Kelly O'Brien, suggest that boomer women will be the first group of women to define their own retirement. "Baby boom women (born between 1946 and 1964) have traversed stages of working girl, working mother and working woman. We will now make the transition to working old woman. We will not replicate the retirement of our mothers. In addition, our life in retirement will be fundamentally different than that of our male counterparts – spouses, brothers, bosses. The reasons are found in our work histories, our demographic profiles and in the basic fact that we continue to be society's caregivers. These factors are intersecting with existing retirement mechanisms, which have not accommodated women's long-term security needs, which are now shaping our future."[60]

Amen.

Things You Can Do As A Boomer Woman Change Agent:

• The recognition that women's unpaid work must receive value towards pensionable benefits is paramount. There are already community groups who work on caregiving issues or pension issues. If you are in one or can contact such a group, do so with a view to making this a goal in addition to the other equity issues they support. There are numerous experts who can help work towards this goal – women friendly lawyers, tax advisers and pension experts. Remember Tupperware? It started in women's living rooms and grew exponentially.

• Another requirement to work for is that of an up-to-three-year dropout period in the CPP to allow caregiving to a needful elder as is now available for parents with small children. More and more midlife boomer women will face this need.

• Keep an eye open for any changes to the present retirement and/or pension system. Find out what any such changes would mean for mid-life women. After all, there are bird watcher groups, so why not pension-watchers?

- Find out all there is to know about your present work situation, whether you are in an employer or occupational pension plan (RPP), what its benefits are, if there are survivor's benefits, if it is a defined benefit or defined contribution plan, and if it will provide a cost-of-living allowance.

- If you live with a spouse or partner, talk about whether there is a will, property arrangements or investments. Find out about your future financial expectations. While this is sometimes hard to talk about, it should not be left for a crisis.

References

1. Compiled from *Women in Canada: A Gender Based Statistical Report*, 5th Ed., (Ottawa: Ministry of Industry, 2006); *The Daily*, Statistics Canada, April 6, 2005 (Cat.no 89-503-XPE); Katherine Marshall, "Converging Gender Roles," Perspectives on Labor and Income, Statistics Canada, (Cat.no.75-001-XIE, 2006): 5-17.

2. Statistics Canada, Income and earnings trends. Table A1.1b. http://www.statcan.ca/english/research/85-570-XIE/2006001/tables/tablea1-1htm.

3. Monica Townson, "Workshop on Family and Gender," *Symposium on New Issues in Retirement* (Ottawa, September 5-6, 2003). Permission to cite by personal communication, August 30, 2005.

4. Monica Townson, "New Vulnerable Groups and living standards in Retirement years" in *New Frontiers of Research in Retirement*. ed. Leroy O. Stone, Statistics Canada (Ottawa: Ministry of Industry, 2006, Cataogue no. 75-001-XIE): 356-357.

5. Doreen Duschene, "More Seniors at Work" in *Perspectives on Labor and Income*, Statistics Canada, February 2004: 15 passim.

6. *Vancouver Sun*, December 9, 2004.

7. *National Post*, July 17, 2002.

8. *Convergence of Male and Female Patterns of Employment Activity*, Statistics Canada, November 25, 2004,<http://www.statcan.gc.ca/pub/11f0024m/pdf/papers-etudes/42249098-eng.pdf>.

9. Anne Marie Ambert, "Divorce: Facts, Causes and Consequences,"Vanier Institute of the Family, <http://www.vifamily.ca/library/cft/divorce.html> (accessed March 24, 2005).

10. Statistics Canada, *The Daily*, May 4, 2004.

11. Sarah Treleaven, "Sixty and Starting Over: Rise in Grey Divorce as Boomers call it Quits" *Financial Post*, April 05, 2008 <http://www.canada.com./topics/news/story.html?id=7cbc596-0273-457d-829d-a2a38712> (accessed May 16, 2008).

12. Andre Bedard and Chris Li, *Death of a Spouse: The Impact on Income for Senior Men and Women*, Analytical Paper, Statistics Canada (Ottawa: Income Statistics Division, Cat..No.11-621-MIE, 2006).

13. *Poverty Profile 2002 and 2003*, National Council of Welfare Reports, (Canada Ministry of Public Works and Government Services, 2006).

14. *Income in Canada*, Statistics Canada, Table "Persons in low income before tax, by prevalence in percent" (2002 to 2006), Catalogue no: 75-202-XIE (2008).

15. *National Post*, February 29, 2004.

16. Lynn McDonald and Leslie A. Robb, QSEP Research Report No. 384 (Hamilton, ON: Research Institute for Quantitative Studies in Economics and Population, Faculty of Social Sciences, McMaster University, 2003).

17. *Vancouver Sun*, January 17, 2005.

18. Judith Treas and Shumpa Mazumadar, "Kinkeeping and Caregiving: Contributions of Older People in Immigrant Families," *Journal of Comparative Studies* 35 (Winter 2004): 107.

19. Catherine Ward-Griffin and Victor W. Marshall, "Reconceptualizing the Relationship Between 'Public' and 'Private' Eldercare," *Journal of Aging Studies* 17 (2003): 189-208.

20. Anne Martin-Matthews, Plenary Address, Canadian Association of Gerontology (Victoria, BC), October 23, 2004. Cited with permission from the author.

21. Susan A. McDaniel, "Women's Changing Relations to the State and Citizenship," *Canadian Review of Sociology and Anthropology* 39, 2 (2002): 126.

22. Malika Hamdad, "Valuing Households' Unpaid Work in Canada 1992-1998: Trends and Sources of Change," *Statistics Canada Economic Conference*, May 2003: 1-14.

23. Katherine Marshall, "Converging Gender Roles," *Perspectives on Labor and Income*, Statistics Canada (Catalogue no. 75-001-XPE, July 2006).

24. <http://swz.salary.com/momsalarywizard/htmls/mswl_momcenter.html>.

25. "Child Care in Sweden: Fact Sheet," The Swedish Institute, 2001.

26. Ward-Griffin and Marshall, Op cit.

27. *Caring for an Aging Society,* Statistics Canada, General Social Survey Cycle 16: 2002, Cat.no.89-583-XIE (Ottawa: Ministry of Industry, 2003).

28. Kelly Cranswick and Donna Dosman."Eldercare: What we know today" Components of Statistics Canada. *Canadian Social Trends*. Cat.no.11-008-X. 2008.

29. Ibid, CST Table 1.

30. Frida Furman, *Facing the Mirror: Older Women and Beauty Shop Culture* (New York and London: Routledge, 1997), 131.

31. Wendy Pyper, "Balancing Career and Care," *Perspectives on Labor and Income*, Statistics Canada (Catalogue no.75-001-XIE: 5-25, November 2006).

32. Ibid., 5: For a comprehensive study on caregiving in Canada which looks, among other considerations, at women caregivers and the value of that work, see Janice Keefe and Beth Rajnovich "To Pay or Not to Pay: Examination Underlying Principles in the Debate on Financial Support for Family caregivers," *Canadian Journal on Aging*, Vol.26 Supplement 1 (2007).

33. Moline, A., "Panel Plans to Send More Tax Dollars to Wall Street," January 28, 2002 <http://womensnews.org/article/cfm/dyn/aid/797/context/archive> (accessed July 13, 2003). See also, "Financial Security For Women Seniors in Canada," Canadian Association of Social Workers (2007).

34. Donald Raymond, "Pension investment board both prudent and responsible," *Vancouver Sun*. November 20, 2006. Please note: Elsewhere the three tiers are differently addressed, calling Tier 1 public pensions; Tier two earnings related public/private, and including RPP's, RRSP's, and likely the CPP. Tier three is alluded to more as private, including investments, insurance, equities, and property. I refer to Tier Two as the CPP and Tier Three as RRSP's etc., as more generally understood in Canada.

35. Canada Pension Plan Benefit rates, Winter 2008, Human Resource Development Canada, Table 3.

36. Service Canada, Old Age Security (OAS) and Payment Rates, January-March 2008, <http://www.hrsdc.gc.ca/en/isp/oas/oasrates.shtml>.

37. *The Daily*, Pension plans in Canada as of January 1 2007, Statistics Canada, <http://www.statcan.ca/Daily/English/080704/td0080704htm> (accessed July 4, 2008).

38. Statistics Canada, "Proportion of labor force and paid workers covered by a registered pension plan (RPP)," Pension Plan in Canada and Labor Force Survey, Last modified 2008-07-08.

39. Monica Townson, R*educing Poverty Among Older Women: The Potential of Retirement Incomes Policies* (Ottawa, Status

of Women Canada, 2000): 28.

40. Yukon Bureau of Statistics, RRSP Contributions, Median RRSP Contributions by Gender 2005 <http://www.eco.gov.yk.ca/stats/>.

41. Statistics Canada, 2008. "Registered retirement savings plan contributions, 2007." Table R-03, Sex, RRSP Contributors 2007. Small Ares and Administrative Data Division, Statistics Canada Catalogue No.17C0006. http://www.statcan.ca/bsolc/English/bsolc?catno+17C0 006.

42. Rene Morissette and Yuri Ostrovsky, *Pension Coverage and Retirement Savings of Canadian Families 1986-2003*, Statistics Canada (Catalogue no. 11F0019MIE-no.286, 2006): 13.

43. National Council of Welfare Reports: 10 passim op.cit.See also Family portrait:*Continuity and change in Canadian families and households in 2006:* National Portrait. *Census families for low income persons before and after tax.* <http://12.statcan.ca/english census06/analysis/famhouse/cenfam/a.cfm> (Accessed 10/25/2007)

44. Monica Townson, *Growing Older,Working Longer:The New Face of Retirement* (Ottawa: Canadian Centre for Policy Alternatives, 2006).

45. Distribution of Retirement Pensions by Age and by Gender, Tables 10 and 11, *Canada Pension Plan and Old Age Security - Monthly Statistical Bulletins*, April 2008.

46. Katherine Marshall, "Incomes of Younger Retired Women: The Past 30 Years," *Perspectives on Labor and Incomes* 12, 4 (Statistics Canada, Catalogue no. 75-001, Winter 2000): 9-17.

47. Lynn McDonald, *The Invisible Retirement of Women, Research on Social and Economic Dimensions of an Aging Population* (SEDAP), Research Paper No.69 (2002): 44.

48. *Vancouver Sun*, September 13, 2004. See also: Marcel Merette, "The Bright Side," Choices, IRPP March 2002 Vol.8. no.1; Robert Brown, "Paying for Canada's Aging Population: How Big is the Problem?" (Toronto, Canadian Institute of Actuaries, March 2002), cited in Townson, 2006.

49. *Vancouver Sun*, March 28, 2006.

50. "Age at Retirement by Sex," Statistics Canada, http://www.statcan.gc.ca/pub/71-222-x/2008001/sectionm/m-age-eng.htm.> (accessed 2/12/2009).

51. Jonathan Chevreau, "Boomers Lucky to Retire by 65," *National Post*, February 17, 2004, 1N1.

52. Lillian Zimmerman et al., "Unanticipated Consequences: A Comparison of Expected and Actual Retirement Timing among Older Women," *Journal of Women and Aging* (2000), 109-28.

53. "The Changing Face of Canadian Workplaces," Canadian Federal Labor Standards Review, 2004 <http://www.fls-ntf.gc.ca/en/bg-01.asp> (accessed April 3, 2006).

54. Leroy O. Stone, Editor in Chief, *New Frontiers of Research on Retirement* (Ottawa: Statistics Canada, Ministry of Industry, Cat. No.75-511-XPE,2006).

55. Ibid., 153.

56. Op.cit., Townson, *Growing Older, Working Longer*: 24.

57. Statistics Canada, *The Daily*, Study: Participation of older workers, 2006, <http://www.statcan.caDaily/English/070824/td070824.htm>.

58. Carolyn J. Rosenthal et al., "Changes in Work and Family over the Life Course: Implications for Economic Security of Today's and Tomorrow's Older Women," *Independence and Economic Security in Old Age*, ed. Frank T. Denton,

Deborah Fretz and Byron G. Spencer (Vancouver, BC: UBC Press, 2000), 108.

59. McDonald, *Invisible Retirement*, 43.

60. Dailey, N. and K. O'Brien, "Baby Boom Women: The Generation of Firsts," in *Women Confronting Retirement: A Nontraditional Guide*. ed. N. Bauer-Maglin and A. Radosh (New Brunswick: J.H.Rutgers University Press, 2003): 150.

Chapter Five

The New Grandparenting:
More than just doting

Grandma lives at the airport

— (eight-year-old)

"Erase the image of grandpa in his rocker on the porch with grandma sitting nearby knitting baby booties while nursing a cup of tea. That was your parents' grandparents."[1] So reads a newspaper report about boomer grandparents. Major changes have certainly occurred to the grandparent role, a fact that is nicely illustrated by an event known as "Grandma's Run" that occurs annually in Markham, Ontario. Sarah Jane Grow, writing about this event, says, "For me, it is theory in action . . . to write here about grandparenting and intergenerational relationships."[2] The organizers invite residents of a nearby care home, most of whom are women, to participate in a program of picnics, barbecues, and sports. Grow reports that one eighty-nine-year-old woman was surrounded by her family, which consists of two daughters, five grandchildren, and eight great-grandchildren; great-grandson James, aged twelve, told Grow that his great-grandmother was "really cool." David Johnston, writing in the *Vancouver Sun*, June 14/08, notes that grandparents are now joining family vacations. Johnston tells us that in the US this is now a 'wildcard', with one third of travel now including either a grandchild, a grandparent or both.

Instead of being an anomaly, such occasions are appearing more regularly on mid-life boomer women's roadmaps, and they will continue to pop up because they are illustrative of the changes wrought by increased longevity and expanded generations, with sometimes four or five generations living in the same time-space. Susan McDaniel, speaking to the 2003 annual meeting of the Canadian Association of Gerontology, coined the term "generationing" to refer to the interactions among these different cohort ages – interactions made largely possible by women's longer life expectancy.[3] Some midlife women are already grandparents and more soon will be, and given the new stages of life occupied by boomer women, being a grandmother will most likely appear on their roadmaps at some point. Even Barbie and Ken have grandparent dolls! In fact, there is already a word which refers to this dynamic: "grandboomers."

The topic of grandparenting is one filled with affection and humor, as witnessed in these comments from a class of eight-year-olds:

- Grandparents are a lady and a man who have no little children of her own. They like other people's.
- A grandfather is a man grandmother.
- Usually grandmothers are fat, but not too fat to tie your shoes.
- They wear glasses and funny underwear.
- They can take their teeth and gums out.
- Grandparents don't have to be smart.
- Asked where his grandma lives, one boy replies, "Oh, she lives at the airport, and when we want her we just go get her. Then when we're done having her visit, we take her back to the airport."

And here are a few from grandparents:

- On the seventh day, God rested. His grandchildren must have been out of town.

- My grandkids believe I'm the oldest thing in the world. After a few hours with them I believe it too.

- The quickest way to get any kid's attention is to sit down and look comfortable.

Grandparents, particularly grandmothers, have traditionally provided caregiving to their grandchildren. This is hardly breaking news, but the present and changing contexts are. The lives of current grandparents are very different than those of previous generations, the most immediate of whom experienced the economic hardships of the Great Depression of the 1930s. In addition, a number of present day grandfathers and some grandmothers fought in the Second World War, which profoundly marked their lives. Litwak et al, social analysts outlining the macro social changes experienced by both baby boomers and their parents, includes economic depression, occupational downsizing, war, and the threat of war.[4] To this list I would certainly add the influx of women into the paid work force. And given restructuring, downsizing, redundancy and economic downturns, many boomer families – though spared a Great Depression and a world war – can be described as facing or having faced a number of recessions or mini-depressions.

However, while it is important to recognize these macro events as the context within which boomer families live, a number of less dramatic events concerning changing grandparenthood also deserve attention. For one thing, as Neena Chappell and her colleagues tell us, more and more people are becoming grandparents, and for longer periods. "At the current time, three quarters of Canadians aged sixty-five years and over have at least one grandchild and most have more than one."[5] These writers remind us, however, that this picture may change; with lower fertility rates and women having children later in life, future older people may be less likely to be grandparents. Interestingly, Litwak et al point out that the increase in longevity implies that today's grandparents may expect to live almost half their lives in that role. This is especially true for grandmothers because women live longer than men.

Other factors in this equation are the changed circumstances of grandmothers' lives. Candace Kemp, writing in *The Social and Demographic Contours of Contemporary Grandparenting*, finds that women's increased participation in the labor force, marital dissolution and the availability of contraception have all contributed to declining birth rates in Canada and other western countries during the twentieth century.[6] This is reflected in such changed forms as single grandmothers, primary grandparents – meaning those who legally adopt or become guardians to grandkids, and what is referred to as "beanpole" families – the lengthening of generations in concert with lower fertility and consequently fewer grandchildren. As well, there are the growing numbers of older grandparents who now have adult grandchildren. These events are among the evolving contours of the new grandparenting. Also important in the changing dynamics of grandmothering are the large numbers of midlife women now in the paid labor force.

Grandma, What Big Roles you Have!

Surprisingly, the question of grandmothers who are in the paid workforce and the relation between that work and their roles as caregivers to grandchildren does not appear to be capturing much interest or attention. Candace Kemp says that "while employment and grandparenthood have typically intersected for men, women's growing labor force participation increases the likelihood that grandmothers will also have work-related roles. This is, of course, more true for younger grandparents, and for those who must work in their later years due to financial necessity."[7] In other words, men have always grandparented while they were part of the paid work force, but now women-that is, midlife boomer women – are also doing paid work while they are grandparenting. In a critique of previous grandmother studies, Nazil Baydar and Jeanne Brooke-Gunn, writing about the situation in the US, found that little is known about grandmother caregiving, particularly caregiving that is not regarded as primary care.[8] They also found that few studies have considered the roles of grandmothers in providing care for other members of the family, in employment and in the community, noting that 35% of the grandmothers in their study were currently employed.

Sarah Arber in another article looks at the grandmother role from a different perspective.[9] She notes the expansion of paid employment for women and lack of available and affordable childcare, discussing the involvement of grandparents providing child care for grandchildren on a regular basis. She suggests daughters (and daughters in law) who have to work full-time for financial reasons, but who do not earn sufficient money to pay for child care, are likely to engage their mothers in routine grandchild care. She states "Thus, working class women in mid and later life are more likely to have their lives constrained by grandparenting than are middle class women." Much more needs to be learned about this grandmother dynamic which may appear, or is already appearing on many boomer women's roadmaps.

We are thus left with many squares missing in the patchwork quilt of what it means to be a midlife boomer grandmother and how women fit grandmothering into their multi-tasking lives. The neglect of attention to the co-relation between grandmothers' paid and unpaid work indicates a gap in present knowledge. A 2002 study by the American Association of Retired Persons (AARP) found that approximately 15% of their respondents provided childcare services for their grandchildren while their parents were at work.[10] An appendix to this report indicated that 17% of their sample were baby boomer age grandparents, born between 1946 and 1964, and that 33% of grandboomers interviewed were male and 67% were female. The majority of these grandboomers (69%) were employed: 53% full-time, 8% part-time and 8% self-employed.[11] Though these figures for working grandboomers are not gendered, at least these researchers were considering current boomer grandparents in relation to their paid work.

Turning to Canadian studies does not provide much more help. According to Canadian researchers Rosenthal and Gladstone, writing in 2004, note that there is a lack of information on how the grandparent role varies when grandparents are employed versus not employed.[12] They placed particular emphasis on grandmothers, and as already noted, 76% of Canadian women aged forty-five to fifty-four and 46% of those aged fifty-five to sixty-four were in the paid workforce in 2004, in addition to the 73% of women with children under sixteen who also had jobs. It would therefore be very interesting to find out how they manage childcare.

Given the apparent lack of Canadian studies of grandboomers – both the younger and older cohorts – in relation to their work and other roles, a number of questions must be asked. How many Canadian grandmothers who are in the paid workforce also act as caregivers to their grandchildren? How many do "double caregiving" to grandchildren, spouses and aging parents? What is the duration of care – short-term, long-term – and how many hours, days, weeks, or months are involved? Have any of them retired specifically for this purpose? What are the costs to them financially, socially and emotionally? What is their marital status and what role does gender play?

A study, released in 2008 (see Chapter 4) found that 57% of Canadian caregivers aged forty-five and over were also in the paid workforce, with women being the majority. As the study states "Caregivers aged 45-54 were at the age where they still had children living at home." Others also juggles employment with family and eldercare tasks as more than half of these caregivers (57%) were employed.[13] It has yet to be established how many in this category were grandboomers, and the nature of that experience. Here are some of the things we do know.

A Kodak Moment: Snapshots of Canadian Grandparenthood

• In 2001 there were 5.7 million Canadian grandparents. Each grandparent had an average of 4.7 grandchildren.

• Only 2% of women and 1% of men forty-five and under were grandparents. In the fifty-five to sixty-five age group, nearly two-thirds of women and just over one-half of men were grandparents.

- About 80% of senior women aged sixty-five and older were grandmothers, while 74% of senior men were grandfathers.

- More than one-half (53%) of all grandparents were married, while 18% were widowed. An additional 10% were divorced or separated or had always been single, while 4% were living common-law.[14]

And widening the lens:

Like so many of the other changing dynamics of family life, grandparenting is far from static.

- Most older Canadians (76% of those aged sixty-five and older) have grandchildren, and most have more than one. Most older Canadians have children, and therefore have the potential to become grandparents.

- First-time grandparenting is now a mid-life event rather than a late-life one.

- Today's grandparents, especially grandmothers, live longer and experience a longer duration of grandparenthood than did their counterparts at the turn of the last century.

- Most young children in North America have grandparents. In 1991, over 90% of ten-year-olds had at least one living grandparent. The likelihood of an individual at age sixty having a surviving grandparent increased from 8% for people born in 1910 to 16% for those born in 1930, and it is predicted to rise to 60% for those born in the 1960s.

- Stepgrandparenthood – becoming a grandparent through divorce or death and subsequent remarriage in either the grandparent or parent generation – has not been studied to any great degree.[15]

Ages and Stages

The timing of grandparenthood is a very important factor in the experience, as is the grandparent's age at the time. This is something grandparents can't control, a reality expressed in an amusing greeting card that reads: "John and Mary wish to announce that they have decided to become grandparents next June." However, it is important to think of both the age of grand-parents and of grandchildren when considering their relationship. In *Grandparenthood in Canada*, Rosenthal and Gladstone point out that there are three significant life stages that need to be taken into account when looking at grandparent-grandchild interaction: "the time when grandchildren are infants and small children, when grandchildren are in later childhood or are young teenagers and when grandchildren are older teenagers and adults."[16] These analysts also note that Canadian couples typically become grandparents in their late forties or early fifties and are thus in their boomerhood. A Canadian expert on the subject, Ingrid Connidis, notes that "about half of all grandparents are under the age of sixty, which has important implications for the type of relationship that is possible between grandparents and their grandchildren."[17] The midlife age (forty-five to sixty-four) at which adults become grandparents has remained constant over the last hundred years, although one generally conjures up images of older grandparents having teen-age grandsons (and some granddaughters) with shaved heads and multi-colored six-inch Mohawks (bright orange seems to be a favourite) as well as lip, ear, and tongue piercings. (I forego describing piercings in other more intimate bodily locations.) But this topic of ages and stages can play out rather curiously. For example, in my seventies,

I already had a grandson attending university while two close friends, both only five years younger than I, had grandkids under the age of one year. This made for some curious phone conversations as I talked to them about my grandson's experiences at university while they described their grandbabies' colic or teething.

The question of the frequency of contact between grandparents and their grandkids is important in these relationships. Rosenthal et al found that the majority of grandparents have regular if not frequent contact with their grandchildren. They further note that the contacts vary with both the ages of the grandchildren and the ages of the grandparents. Geographic proximity, of course, also plays a role. For example, of Canadian adult grandchildren over age fifteen with a grandparent still living, 39% saw their grandparent more than once a month, while 41% saw her/him less than once a month.[18] Technology has certainly made it possible for more regular contact. The AARP grandparent report found that 65% of grandparents had telephone contact with grandchildren at least once a week, with lesser numbers using e-mail. The Internet affords contact both from home and from work, with 48% of those interviewed using it from home.[19] In the past grandmothers showed the newest baby's picture in a "Grandma's Brag Book"; now grandmothers are more likely to use a palm pilot or a blackberry or ipod. There are many, though, who find themselves technologically challenged. A former Canadian federal minister of justice, Irwin Cotler, told this story on himself: his three-year-old grandson approached to ask him if he could help fix the VCR. Mr.Cotler replied that he was not good at doing that sort of thing, whereupon his grandson replied impatiently, "I know that, Grandpa. I just want you to hold me up so I can fix it." One of my focus group women who is in her nineties reported that while on a cruise she had e-mailed her grandkids quite regularly until she found out the cost, at which time she reverted to her own generations' standby-postcards.

Meanings and Values

Grandparents are uniquely placed to transmit family values. Please note that my use of this term "family values" has nothing to do with the current right-wing fundamentalist usurpation of it, as this faction resists the more liberal views evolving as family dynamics change. I use the term "family values" to refer to the belief systems and notions of morality passed by grandparents from one generation of a family to the next and, now that generations are expanding, to more than one. As Rosenthal and Gladstone point out, "grandparents . . . pass down history, traditional family and social values, act as confidants and role models."[20] In its grandparenting report AARP also found that grandparents thought that teaching grandchildren values, telling them about their family history and teaching them about religion and spirituality were important. However, in so doing there are cautions which apply, according to Rona Stovall Hanks who cites four areas of responsibility to which she gives equal weight: knowing how to be a grandparent while leaving parenting to the child's parents; being strong for the grandchild, especially in holding to family values and morality; providing family stability for the child and serving as a role model.[21] In a survey Hanks conducted she asked, "What is most important in your relationship with grandchildren?" Seventy-eight percent of respondents said it was their ability to influence their grandchildren's values. But while this may be an admirable goal, it is important that such influence not be overbearing and not conflict with parents' or older grandchildren's values.

This is not to suggest that all, or even most, grandparent relations are of the Hallmark, tension-free type. Grandparent experiences are not homogeneous. One older woman in one of my focus groups stated clearly, "I told my daughter I am not a baby-sitting grandmother," and this no doubt reflects the feeling of others. One anecdote about a grandboomer who is in her late fifties and lives in Toronto is instructive in this regard. She is a single parent, a professional who is divorced and who has custody of her teen-aged son. Unfortunately, he did not show much aptitude for school, for getting a job or, for that matter, anything else except an ability to reproduce. At age sixteen, he and his fifteen-year-old girlfriend were expecting a baby. The girlfriend came from a dysfunctional family, and also had few skills. Because the young mother's parents were incapable, and because she didn't want her grandchild in a foster home, it fell to this grandboomer to house her son's family, support them and take responsibility for her grandchild's needs. Fortunately, her profession allowed her to work a great deal out of her home. Clearly, there is much to be learned about grandboomers and the circumstances that can generate their unpaid caregiving. None of these considerations negate the kind of giving that midlife boomers in turn offer their parents when the latter are frail or otherwise in need.

Gender and Grandparenting: A Unisex Future?

The fact that there are gender differences in the ways men and women experience grandparenting is hardly a surprise. Two observers, Glenda Spitz and Russell Ward, note that gender is an organizing feature of many family roles and relationships. They point out that "this is reflected in intergenerational relations between parents and adult children as well as between grandparents and grandchildren, including stronger ties and bonds along the female lines."[22] They argue that, as with caregiving in general, the activities of grandmothers and grandfathers reflect traditional gender roles, "with grandfathers engaging in instrumental activities and grandmothers in 'warmer' more expressive activities."[23]

These long held views may be on the cusp of change in the context of the many social and demographic shifts taking place. Living longer than men, more will be single grandmothers and may also participate in a greater range of intergenerational activities. However, the fact that the gap in male-female longevity is slowly closing could mean that more men will also be grandparents for longer periods.

The mother-daughter bond also appears to significantly influence grandparental gender relations. In North America, according to Rosenthal and Gladstone, the mother-daughter tie tends to be stronger than any other parent-child ties. Other observers have reflected on the mother/ daughter role and the belief that maternal grandparents play a more influential role in grandchildren's lives than paternal grandparents. There is some evidence to suggest that adolescent grandchildren feel closer to their maternal grandparent than to their paternal grandparent, and that the maternal grandmother is key in terms of feelings of closeness.[24] One woman in the focus groups I conducted in preparation for this book, a woman in her seventies, put it this way: "Whenever I was in trouble or was going through a rough time, I knew I could usually talk about it to my [maternal] grandmother. She always made me feel better." This appears to be a fairly common observation.

What about grandfathers? Demographic and familial evolution is having an important effect on grandfathering. Spitz and Ward put it nicely when they wrote that "grandfathers have been considered the 'forgotten men' in the family as the maternal and expressive nature of grandparenting is presumed to make grandfather a peripheral role."[25] However, as men are also living longer, though not yet as long as women, and as they retire, they are getting a chance to respond directly to intergenerational changes. Also, there is an opportunity for mid-life or older grandfathers, watching how some of today's fathers are more involved than they were in childrearing, to see that grandfathering provides a second chance. Indeed, there seems to be a trend towards unisex roles. And as Spitz and Ward point out, a decrease in role differentiation "implies that grandmothers and grandfathers would relate to grandchildren in increasingly similar ways as they age and as other life roles become more similar."[26] This is indeed a welcome development. I talked to an active, retired grandfather who told me that he and his wife, also retired, consider themselves to be engaged in co-grandparenting, together doing many things with their grandkids including traveling, hiking, and skiing. He and his wife are careful to minimize gender roles; for example, he does half the cooking in their everyday lives anyway so their grandkids simply see this as a given. As this is an educated, middle-class couple, they may be somewhat atypical, but this may not be for long.

Another aspect of grandmothering which needs more attention is that of lesbian grandparenting. An American study conducted by Dorothy Whelan et al notes that, despite the increasing attention being given to grandparenting, there is a void in the gerontological research on lesbian, gay, bisexual, and transgendered (LGBT) grandparent-grandchild relations. They find that the sexual orientation of the grandparent is seldom considered.[27] These authors say that their work, which was published in 2000, is the first study of lesbian grandmothers and they found, to no one's surprise, that there is an assumption that all grandparents are heterosexual. Carefully stressing that their sample was not representative or generalizable, they go on to describe the grandmother role from the viewpoint of nine lesbian grandmothers between the ages of thirty-five and sixty-four. These women saw their grandmother role much as do heterosexual grandmothers and emphasized providing emotional support to grandchildren (and their parents) and enjoying time with them, a perception of grandmothering that is remarkably similar to the predominant companionate type of straight grandparents.

An investigation by Nancy Orel and Christine Fruhauf, both more recent and more complex than that of Whelan et al, concentrates on the effect of the grandmothers' lesbian and bisexual orientation on their relations with their grandchildren.[28] Again, a relatively small number of women was studied: sixteen, of whom twelve identified as lesbian and four as bisexual. The majority of these grandmothers were in a partnered relationship. From this study, they extrapolate that from the estimated three million lesbian and gay parents in the United States, one to two million are, or will be, grandparents, but they found that these grandmothers' roles and motivations were similar to those of heterosexual grandmothers.

A difference did emerge, however, between those grandmothers who were "out" and those who had not disclosed their sexual orientation to their adult children and/or grandchildren. Twelve of the sixteen women had "come out" to their children. Those who had not were uncomfortable and stressed about hiding their sexual orientation. Among their reasons for remaining in the closet were concerns about how their grandchildren would react to their being lesbian or bisexual. One of the closeted grandmothers noted humorously that if she disclosed her sexual orientation, her granddaughter would be more upset to know that her grandmother was still having sex (and would consider it gross) than she would be to know that her grandmother was a lesbian. All sixteen women agreed that, while their sexual orientation should not matter, our culture makes it matter. The majority reported that their relationships with their adult children, particularly with their adult daughters, often determined their roles as grandmothers. This relationship either facilitated or discouraged an emotional bond between a grandmother and her grandchildren. Managing the disclosure of their sexual orientation was, therefore, a primary issue.

Generationing: Adult Grandchildren.

The fact that grandparents are living longer allows them to graduate from activities with younger grandkids, whose energy is apparently inexhaustible and can be tiring, to affiliations with adult grandchildren on a mature basis. "In fact," as Candace L. Kemp notes in a study that looks at the relationships between grandparents and adult grandchildren, "most grandparents and grandchildren will experience at least twenty years of inter-generational overlap and in many cases their lives will overlap for thirty, possibly even forty years or more."[29] Such startling possibilities are hard to absorb except for grandparents already involved with adult grandchildren, but they clearly attest to the changing social stages of women's lives and to a lesser degree, men's. Relations themselves evolve and change as both grandparents and grandchildren go through varied life events – for example, a grandparent's health problems or a granddaughter or grandson becoming involved in a relationship or planning to marry. One light-hearted anecdote related to me concerned a grandmother who had always praised her grandson for his achievements, encouraging him to do more, even being on the sidelines during his sports activities, shouting with the parents "Way to go!" as current parental practice dictates. One day she was put to the test when he arrived on her doorstep, aged sixteen and waving his hours-old driver's licence, and invited her to go for a first drive. Despite the apprehension that she kept carefully hidden, she accepted the invitation and they both survived: one small example of how relations with a maturing grandchild may develop.

As they become adults, grandchildren may come to appreciate the social contexts of their grandparents' lives. Grandparents' "stories" may eventually be recognized as providing context to the socio-economic and emotional realities of grandparents' lived lives. My own ears were closed and I suffered impatiently through my late mother's oft-repeated stories about her experience with the Spanish flu, which she contracted during the First World War. Now that the possibility of another worldwide avian flu pandemic hovers, I feel awed by the implications of her stories, which I have now shared with my own grandkids.

It is commonly felt that the golden rule of grandparenthood, at least in Western cultures, is "thou shalt not interfere." Candace Kemp examines this ethic from the perspective of both grandparents and adult grandchildren, and all of the following quotations are taken from her study.[30] One of the participants, a ninety-one-year-old grandmother, said, "I don't think a grandparent should criticize anything about a grandchild even if they think maybe it is not the right thing. Just go along with it." Another grandmother volunteered, "I think it is foolish for grandparents to try and run their grandchildren . . . not only foolish, but sometimes impossible . . . I think some grandparents do try to influence their grandchildren, and I don't think that's fair." And, according to a 32-year-old granddaughter who was discussing grandparent interference, "You take it in stride. They're older and set in their ways and that's how it is. I mean, I just let it go in one ear and out the other . . . they don't necessarily understand my choices; I hope they can appreciate them."

On the topic of respect, Kemp found that her adult grandchildren interviewees were very conscious of negative stereotypes that associate old age with decline and dependence. In the words of a twenty-eight-year-old grandson, "From a sense of respect, I think treating my grandmother as an equal and not thinking that she's weak or frail . . . I don't ever feel sorry for her." The topic of intergenerational reciprocity was expressed in a number of different ways. A twenty-three-year-old grandson put it this way: "I would think that the adult grandchild role might be some sort of, kind of returning, say justifying that they have done everything right . . . Like I look at my relationship with my grandmother and I think the fact that I turned out to be what I consider half decent and that I spend time with her as proof." Despite some reservations, Kemp felt that adult grandchildren wanted grandparents to be involved in their socialization and appeared to have great respect for their grandparents' experiences, to which a number of them referred.

The many changes and shifting family dynamics discussed above and their effects on grandmothering are nicely stated by Michelle A. Miller-Day when she writes "There have been so many extraordinary changes for women in the past century. These changes have shifted cultural and individual ideals of whom one should be as a woman, grandmother, mother, daughter or granddaughter. Women's changing roles in this past century have required women to adapt to these changing ideals."[31]

Case History

My own grandmotherhood occurred when I was a mid-life single parent, and the dynamics of my relations with my oldest grandson may be representative of patterns now developing, given demographic changes and the evolution of less traditional forms of parenting. I worked in an academic institution and had regular but flexible hours; both his parents, my older daughter (a boomer) and her husband, were (and are) in the workforce and appreciated my babysitting and childminding, which also provided them relief from their fast-forward professional lives. My first grandchild's birth was an unexpectedly profound experience for me. I wanted to be with him a great deal. This meant repeating some of the juggling and multi-tasking I had mastered as a single parent. He does not have any siblings, and spent many weekends and overnights with me. I often picked him up from daycare late Friday afternoon. I loved being with him. We had summer stays when he wasn't in camp and we would go to the beautiful Whistler area and take long walks through the trees and alongside streams and lakes.

In addition, being a close-knit family unit, the four of us travelled and did many things together. I retired when this grandson was ten, after which I had more time for him and the grandchildren of my other boomer daughter, whose family circumstances were different and did not require much help from me.

Our activites were appropriate to his ages and stages, and, as he got older, we watched TV, especially cooking shows, which he adored, and went to concerts, movies, museums, libraries, the planetarium, and restaurants. I travelled to Europe with him when he was fifteen. As he started establishing his own interests, which included acting, from time to time I took him to acting lessons, tryouts (or "cattle calls" as they are known), and then to play rehearsals when he got a part. Later, when he got parts in TV commercials, I accompanied him to "shoots" waiting many hours through endless "takes" that sometimes lasted into the night. As he grew older and his life became fuller and richer with study, work, and friends, and as I continued my own professional activities, our times together became less frequent. They were often marked by quirky gifts, for example, when I was on my way to an aging conference, he got me a button that read: "Damn old - any further questions?" Now there are occasional, breathless cell phone calls made from his car (and yes, I cringe but bite my tongue), and when I see him, a tall, sophisticated, self-assured twenty-six-year-old university graduate with a full-time job, he in some ways seems a semi-stranger to me. He has his own world. But this is the existential paradox of a mode of parenting and grandparenting that emphasizes providing children with the ability to make choices, to grow into independence and to develop worlds of their own.

Passing it Forward: Part 1

Continuing with the lifecourse approach – that is, looking at family events as a cumulative process over the course of people's lives – we now come to family occurrences that have serious consequences for both grandparents and grandchildren. Divorce or separation, for example, certainly strains family relationships, while the dysfunctional behavior of adult children may result in more intense grandparenting. As Barbara Hirschorn comments, "Grandparent caregiving stretches, reorganizes and redefines the relationship between family members; redraws the boundaries of family and often of household units and redirects the transfer of resources within the family."[32] In other words, there can be greater grandparent involvement during times of family crises.

Grandparent activities and assistance fall into three categories: occasional help, short-term help, and long-term help.[33] Occasional help can include short emergencies such as taking a sick child for medical attention or relieving the adult parent by child-minding. Or it may involve taking a grandchild to a dentist or other appointments when the parents are unavailable due to work or other commitments.

Short-term help would include looking after a grandchild during its parent's illness or perhaps when the parent is looking for a job or taking further training. It could include looking after the grandchildren for a few weeks while their parents are on holidays. Short-term grandparenting on a fairly regular basis can make it possible for a daughter or son to keep her or his job, although this is a large contribution of time on the part of the grandparent and describing it as "short-term" seems a bit of a stretch. Long-term help includes adopting the parent role (that is, co-parenting), which could include looking after a grandchild for part or all of the working week.

An article by Katrin Kritz on grandmothering refers to "second moms" who fill parents' needs for childcare after mothers return to work, in addition to providing a social and financial safety net for their daughters and grandchildren.[34]

One anecdotal case concerns an older grandmother who looked after a preschool grandchild in the child's home while the parents worked. At lunch time she took the child back to her own home in order to make lunch for her husband and then back to the child's home until the parents returned. It is unlikely that this kind of double caregiving will continue in the new and more enlightened era of grandboomers and of more involved and evolved grandfathers who can surely open a tin of soup or make a tuna sandwich for themselves.

Hopefully, the misbegotten responsibility of this grandmother will fast fade from the grandparenting radar screen.

More demanding occasions occur when grand-parents co-parent or become surrogate parents for the long haul. Rosenthal et al found that since the 1980s there has been an increasing number of grandparents who have taken on a parental role with their grandchildren. Reasons for this include an increase in alcohol and drug abuse, divorce, teen pregnancy, incarceration, and the AIDS epidemic.[35] Other reasons might include the death of an adult or a serious illness. An American investigation by Margaret Jendrek found that grandparents undertake such long-term care arrangements because they want to help the grandchild's parents, they don't want the grandchild in daycare or a sitter's house or they are concerned because the grandchild's mother is working full-time and/or having emotional problems.

Many grandparents are afraid of having a grandchild placed in foster care. In one instance, Jendrek reports that a grandmother who had custody of a grandchild for two years had this to say about her adult daughter: "She would leave Charlie [the grandson] for several days at a time . . . You can't just leave a child for days and days on end and not give them any time when you're going to be back or even give the baby-sitter any time when you're going to be back."[36]

The divorce of adult children plays a significant role in longer term grandparenting. Rosenthal and Gladstone report that "advice to grandparents whose adult child has been separated or divorced, ranged from 'give support', 'be there' to 'don't take sides', 'don't give advice.'"[37] Grandparents can find themselves playing mediating roles, and sometimes a strong mother-daughter bond may lead to friction between the grandparents themselves. The ethic of "non-interference" can also put grandparents in a double bind because the grandchild or grandchildren can look to them for support and assistance when the grandparents are themselves torn.

Another development in family life that involves grandparents is co-residence, with grandchildren and grandparents living in the same household. In Canada this is considered to be a major change in family patterns as they developed over the twentieth century. Now it appears that the number of three generations living under one roof increased by 40% between 1986 and 1996, possibly due to an increase in immigrations from Asia, as many Asians favour multigenerational living arrangements.[38] There is also what is called the "skip generation." In 2001 in Canada, 56 700 grandparents (that is, 1% of all grandparents) were living with their grandchildren without either of the latter's parents being present. These skip grandparents account for about 12% of the grandparents who share households with their grandchildren. Two-thirds of the grandparents in these households are women, and just under one-half (46%) are retired.[39] Grandparents might also live with a divorced or separated adult parent. In such circumstances the grandparent is likely contributing significantly to the finances in addition to caregiving time. Though these Canadian numbers are small at present, we can't predict what the future will bring. It is also too early to assess what, if any, the effect of Canada's decreasing divorce rates (assuming they continue to decline) will have on grandparenting (see discussion on grey divorces in Chapter 4).

Some of the circumstances that affect grand-parenting are unplanned, often amounting to a curve ball thrown at people who did not anticipate parenting a second time around but rather looked forward to a more relaxed existence. These dramatic events can exact a considerable toll on grandparents especially if they have to curtail their lives to become primary caregivers again. One such afflicted grandmother in my focus groups said, "I've done this once already and didn't think I'd have to do it again." It is not an uncommon response. Despite such expressions of understandable resentment, it appears that many grandparents are determined to do what they can to help when such situations arise.

A Canadian Broadcasting Corporation (CBC) documentary on grandparenting in Canada aired on

Newsworld on February 26, 2004, focused on one sixty-five-year-old woman living in Ontario who had worked in a cafeteria most of her life and was looking forward to retirement with her husband. They had two male grandchildren in elementary school, but their daughter was an alcoholic and unable to care for her children. The grandparents took legal custody of the grandchildren because they didn't want them to go into foster care, fearing that the family would lose touch with the children and that they would not be properly brought up. Now, as the filmmaker explained, "Instead of putting their feet up, they were putting boots on their kids," taking them to school, and everywhere else. But worse was to come: the grandfather died, and the grandmother now looks after the kids all on her own. She finds it hard without her husband, and is worried about the future, especially when the boys go to high school. "Sometimes I'm tired at night," she says.

She has used up all her savings, has a mortgage to pay, and is constantly overdrawn at the bank. She also has to pay for a private tutor, as one of the boys has a form of autism. In addition, she pays for karate lessons because she feels that it will help the children gain self-confidence. She has joined an early childhood development group where she can talk to those who are in the same situation. According to the expert consulted for this documentary, the numbers of grandparents raising grandchildren has increased considerably in the last decade, possibly due to the growing use of crack cocaine and higher rates of incarceration.

The dynamics of grandparenting are constantly changing as families themselves change, and we do not know whether the case above describes a situation that will become more common. If it does, then some midlife boomer women will have to navigate a large obstruction on their later lives' roadmaps. It is important to recognize that not all grandparents can or will participate in the same way during family difficulties, especially if their health is poor, if they lack the resources or if they simply don't want to.

Passing it Forward: Part 2

The current crisis interpretation of population aging by some of the-sky-is-falling variety of experts has promulgated mainly negative projections, among them that the growing numbers of older persons will supposedly be a "burden" that the following generations will have to bear. This crisis perspective does not jibe with many realities of older person's lives and conveniently ignores caregiving, which, of course, includes grandparenting. There are more tangible aspects of the intergenerational exchanges between grandparents, their adult children and their grandchildren, that is, the substantive aspects of giving from older generations to the younger ones, specifically financial aid and gift giving. In fact, a global survey conducted by Oxford University's Institute on Ageing, HSBC Securities (Canada) Ltd finds "The study explodes the myth that older people are dependents whose care drains vital resources from nations struggling with aging populations." Commenting on this study, Virginia Galt found the study shows that older people contribute both through their taxes and provide financial support and caregiving to their grandchildren.[40] This study of twenty-two countries included Canada.

Social analyst David Cheal has recognized that grandparents are a Canadian social resource, but he writes that at the same time "the role of grandparents has been largely ignored by social researchers and family policy specialists."[41] However Jason Lian and his co-investigators report that "recent literature has begun to recognize the significant contributions made by seniors to their families and communities and the importance of these contributions to the economy."[42] We are all familiar with anecdotal information about grandparents paying for grandkids music lessons or sports activities, even educational fees but this kind of giving actually occurs on a much larger scale. An American observer suggests that American grandparents should be considered "Heroic Family Contributors." They estimate that, through unpaid supervision and childcare, grandparents provide $17 to $29 billion annually towards the support of their children and grandchildren.[43]

Writing in 2000, Jason Lian et al estimated that, including travel time, the total market value of unpaid help contributed by individuals aged sixty-five and older in Canada was approximately $5.5 billion and that, excluding travel time, it is approximately $4.7 billion. They state that "calculated as a percentage of Old Age Security (OAS) and Guaranteed Income Supplement (GIS) payments, this market value represents 29.3% and 25.2%, respectively. In other words, Canadian seniors aged sixty-five and older returned at least one-quarter of what they received in public pensions in the form of unpaid assistance to others."[44] Stating it in this fashion is indeed an eye-opener. We can safely assume that a significant proportion of these large amounts of unpaid labor involved grandparenting. I suggest that grandparental/grandmother daycare, for example, can be considered an economic transfer in that a grandmother providing even part-time child-minding enables her adult child to get and keep a job, to earn and pay taxes-a clear benefit to the Canadian economy. Another example is that of the adult child who suffers severe financial difficulties, such as losing a job, and comes to live in their parents' or grandparents' basement; this too can be considered an economic transfer. It is well to keep in mind the caution noted by Arber (above) regarding calls on grandmothers of daughters in the paid workforce are, or may be called on for regular childcare.

In a 2004 report, a Canadian study by Ploeg et al focuses on intergenerational financial transfers from older parents to adult children and grandchildren. Again, such features as geographic closeness, marital status, the health of the older parents, the number of children and grandchildren and the available resources all influence the ability of grandparents to give money. Looking through a life-course lens and acknowledging that the participants in their study were all educated and middle-class, Ploeg and her co-investigators found that money was given to adult children for the purchase of a home or cottage or car, for weddings, and as gifts of cash as well as for living and educational expenses. Transfers to grandchildren took the form of trusts or education assistance that ranged from $5000 to $30 000.[45]

These gifts were motivated by love and commitment and by the desire to pass on an early inheritance; by the felt importance of maintaining a history of family giving and by the wish to alleviate financial need during difficult times, such as divorce or bankruptcy. Several persons in this study referred to inter-generational reciprocity as a reason for giving. Among them was a married seventy-seven-year-old man who said, "As a very young couple we were assisted by our parents, and we feel strongly that this is a very strong motive to keep family close and trusting." Similarly, a seventy-nine year-old married grand-mother said, "I carry on how I was helped by my family." Interestingly, some people were motivated to help precisely because they themselves had not received assistance. One sevety-nine-year-old divorced grand-father stated, "I did not receive financial assistance from my father or mother. I wanted to improve [my] children [and] grandchildren's lives." A seventy-six-year-old man recalled hard times: "Born before the Great Depression and living through it, one never forgets total destruction. The suffering my parents went through is forever etched in my mind. Rising through the ashes of destitution, I was determined if an opportunity presented itself, my family would never be exposed to the suffering I went through. I cannot describe the joy of sharing assets with my children, helping them to advance in life." One grandparenting couple commented that generous parents will be equally generous grandparents, assuming they have the appropriate financial resources. Again, it should be noted that not all grandparents are in a position to assist or wish to do so.

I know from a number of talks I have given that whenever I mention the subject of parental and grandparental giving, the heads of my listeners will start to nod vigorously in assent. Of course, the above anecdotal comments come from a generation that, though suffering through both a depression and a war, also had the benefit of the post-war growth of the welfare state in Canada, allowing many to acquire assets such as homes. Midlife boomers contexts are different but assistance to their families likely appears on their roadmaps. In an American Association of Retired Persons (AARP) financial report, which they refer to as Our First-of-its-Kind Research "Grandparents want to Financially Support and Empower Their Grandchildren" the report found that grandparents spend about $600 per year in total on their grandchildren.[46] The typical grandparent, having four grandchildren, means that they spend about $150 per child. With a median income of approximately $46 000, according to this report, the grandparents surveyed typically spent 1.3 of their annual income on their grandkids. Margaret Cruikshank, in her book *Learning to be Old*, captured the response of grandparents to new economic and familial realities when she wrote, "An accurate picture of the transfer of wealth between generations might show aging parents keeping an underemployed son or a jobless daughter afloat in the swirling waters of the global economy."[47] We are left to wonder why the scope of such generous contributions on the part of older Canadian remains largely unheralded.

The future of such intergenerational transfers may be less than certain given cutbacks to social programs that affect both midlife boomers and grandparents. This is a case of short-term (and short-sighted) policy agendas, for example, the paucity of affordable daycare and home care that may have long-term consequences. The evidence of the giving of both time and money and its value to the economy should be kept front and centre as older people continue to be assailed by ageist bigots who claim that they are draining, or will drain, our resources. In fact, without such giving, the public sector might have to be much larger. The social and economic contributions of grandparents and grandboomers should be making headlines.

Gazing into a Crystal Ball: Twenty-five Years into the Future

I grant you that gazing into crystal balls is not a very scientific method, but dreams and imagination, being outside the box, are vital when it comes to envisioning change. Our lives have been transformed hugely over the past quarter century. What might they look like after the next quarter century? For example, let's take a look at what might happen to seniors' centres:

1. There will be no more seniors' centres. In fact, the category "senior citizen" itself will be consigned to

the trash bin of history. Given new sensibilities and changed lives, the word is already an anachronism. There will be centres, but they will be called "maturity centres."

2. Women will still constitute the majority of people in maturity centres, but the age gap between women and men will be much narrowed. Given healthier lifestyles and medical advances, there will be more older men around than there are now. Women's longevity will have reached a plateau, resulting in greater gender balance.

3. Maturity centres will be free-standing, and will have large fitness components, gyms, and exercise rooms. There will be racquet ball, squash and tennis courts and, of course, swimming pools. For the mature, there will be extreme sports such as whitewater rafting and snowboarding.

4. Each maturity centre will have a part-time health component, staffed by a doctor, nurse, therapists and other health care professionals.

5. Each maturity centre will provide daycare, with decently paid daycare workers to accommodate grandparents, many of whom will be in the paid work force.

6. Maturity centres will have their own libraries, which will contain material on a vast range of professional, business, political, and social topics. Computers will be yesterday's news by then, but whatever the case, these centres will have state-of-the-art technology rooms.

7. Programming will be more active at maturity centres than it ever was in senior centres. Buses will still be used, but many members will bicycle to outings, which will include visits to museums and environmental centres, though there will still be trips to Las Vegas.

8. There will be men's support groups, perhaps for grandfathers, widowers, or those who are caregiving their spouses and others.

9. Maturity centres will have maturity advocacy groups (MAGS), which will be nationally organized to act as a powerful lobby on behalf of matures.

10. Maturity centres will also have a part-time travel agency, because members will increase their traveling, taking tours that will meet their mental, physical and spiritual needs.

And why not?

Things You Can Do As A Boomer Woman Change Agent:

- If you are a mid-life boomer providing grandmothering services, you are already a change agent who is providing assistance to your adult children. If you have a spouse who is not similarly involved, help nudge his participation towards more unisex grandparenting.

- Stereotypes of grandparents may be slowly changing, but they still require vigilance. For example, why do newspaper descriptions refer to the fact that the person in the story they are reporting is a grandmother when the story is not about grandparenting? If the reference is irrelevant, let the editors know. Also such references as "the blue rinse set" displays ageism towards grandmothers, that is, unless you know grandfathers who color their hair blue.

- It is important for grandparents to be social and familial historians. Your stories about your own and your grandparents' lives are important learning experiences for grandkids, both historically and as a way to impart the values and beliefs held. (Try not to be repetitive, as this is a major turnoff for grandkids.)

- If you are interactive with your adult grandchildren, it is important to stay current with the things that concern them and use methods of communication relevant to them. Learn to text message, blog, look at YouTube and use Facebook.

- If your own grandparents made positive contributions to your life, think of why this was the case. Avoid the things they did which irritated you.

- There is now a Grandmothers Campaign with over one hundred groups of Canadian grandmothers who help African grandmothers forced to assume the raising of grandchildren, because HIV/AIDS has robbed those children of parents. If this kind of work appeals to you, there is ample information on the net.

References

1. Samantha Critchell, Associated Press, in *Times Colonist*, October 19, 2004.

2. Alexandra Gill, *Vancouver Sun*, May 24, 2003.

3. Susan McDaniel, *Puzzling the Pieces of the Intergenerational: Research and Policy Linkages, with Implications for Education and Practice*, Keynote address, Canadian Association of Gerontology Annual Meeting (Toronto), October 30-November 1, 2003. Permission to cite given by the author.

4. Eugene Litwak et al., "Grandparents and Grandchildren in Family Systems: A Social Development Perspective," *Global Aging and Challenges to Families*, ed. Vern L. Bengston and Ariela Lowenstein (New York: DeGruyter Inc., 2003), 79.

5. Neena Chappell et al., *Aging in Canada*. (Toronto: Prentice Hall, 2003), 298.

6. Candace L. Kemp, "Social and Demographic Contours of Contemporary Grandparenthood: Mapping Patterns in Canada and the United States," *Journal of Contemporary Family Studies* 32, 2 (2003): 189.

7. Ibid., 190.

8. Nazil Baydar and Jeanne Brooks-Gunn, "Profiles of Grandmothers Who Care for their Grandchildren in the United States," *Journal of Family Relations* 47, 4 (1998): 386.

9. Sarah Arber, "Gender and Late Life: Change, Choice and Constraints" in John A. Vincent, Chris R. Phillipson and Murna Downs. Eds. *The Futures of Old Age*. London: Sage Publications, (2006), 57-58.

10. American Association of Retired Persons (AARP), *The Grandparent Study 2002*, Data collected by AARP and prepared by Roper ASW, Curt Davies, with assistance of Dameka Williams <http://research.aarp.org> (accessed October 12, 2005).

11. Ibid., 47.

12. Carol J. Rosenthal and James Gladstone, "Grandparenthood in Canada". Vanier institue of the Family. (2004.) passim.

13. Kelly Cranswick and Donna Dusman. "Eldercare: What we know today." Components of Statistics Canada. *Canadian Social Trends*. Cat.no.11-008-X: 49. 2008.

14. "Grandparenting and Grandchildren," *The Daily*, Statistics Canada, December 9, 2003, <http://www.statcan.ca/Daily/English/031209/d031209b.htm>.

15. Rosenthal and Gladstone, "Grandparenthood in Canada," passim.

16. Rosenthal, 12.

17. Ingrid Arnet Connidis, *Family Ties and Aging* (Thousand Oaks: Sage Publications, 2001), 168.

18. Rosenthal and Gladstone, "Grandparenthood in Canada," 7.

19. AARP, 22. op.cit.

20. Rosenthal and Gladstone, "Grandparenthood in Canada," 2.

21. Rona Stovall Hanks, "Grandma, What Big Teeth You Have: The Social Construction of Grandparents in American Business and Academe," *Journal of Family Issues* 22, 5 (2001): 663.

22. Glenna Spitz and Russell A. Ward, "Gender Variations," *Handbook on Grandparenthood*, ed. Maximiliane E. Szinovacz

(Westport CT: Greenwood Press, 1998), 113.

23. Ibid., 118.

24. Rosenthal and Gladstone, 9.

25. Spitz and Ward, 118.

26. Ibid., 115.

27. Dorothy M. Whelan, Jerry J. Bigner and Clifton E. Barber, "The Grandmother Role as Experienced by Lesbian Women," *Journal of Women and Aging* 12, 33/4 (2002).

28. Nancy A. Orel and Christine A. Fruhauf, "Lesbian and Bisexual Grandmothers' Perception of the Grandparent-Grandchild Relationship," *Journal of Gay, Lesbian, Bisexual, and Transgender Family Studies* 2, 1 (2006): 43-70. See also D. Kimmel, T. Rose, & S. David (Eds.) *Research and Clinical Perspectives on Lesbian, Gay, Bisexual and Transgender Aging*. (New York: Columbia Press), 248-274.

29. Candace L. Kemp."Grand Expectations: The Experience of Grandparents and Adult Grandchildren". Canadian Journal of Sociology. 29, 4, (2004) p.500.

30. ibid. passim.

31. Michelle A. Miller-Day, *Communication Among Grandmothers, Mothers and Adult Daughters: A Qualitative Study of Maternal Relationships*, (London: Lawrence Erlbaum Associates, Publishers, 2004), 137.

32. Barbara A. Hirshorn, "Grandparents as Caregivers" in *Handbook on Grandparenthood*, ed. Maxamilliane E. Szinovacz (Westport CT: Greenwood Press, 1998): 202. See also Margaret Platt "Grandparents who Parent Their Grandchildren: Circumstances and Decisions" Gerontologist 34, 2, (1994): 200-16.

33. Ibid., 201.

34. Katrin Kritz, "How Grandmothers Become Second Moms: Policies and Grandmothering in Britain, Germany and Sweden," *Journal for the Association of Mothering* 7-2 (Fall/Winter 2005): 49-62.

35. Rosenthal and Gladstone, 2.

36. Margaret Platt Jendrek, "Grandparents Who Parent Their Grandchildren: Circumstances and Decisions," The Gerontologist 34, 2 (1994): 210.

37. Rosenthal and Gladstone, 7.

38. Ellen Gee and Barbara A. Mitchell, "One Roof: Exploring Multi-Generational Households in Canada," *Voices: Essays on*

Canadian Families, ed. Marion Lynn, 2nd Ed., (Toronto: Nelson Thompson Learning, 2003), 292.

39. "Grandparents and Grandchildren 2001," Statistics Canada, *The Daily*, December 9, 2003. <www.statcan.ca/Daily/English/031209/d031209b.htm> (accessed January 14, 2005).

40. Virginia Galt, "Older Workers a drain? Not a chance, study finds," *The Globe and Mail*, May 23, 2007.

41. David Cheal, "Introduction: Contextualizing Demographic Concerns," in *Aging and Demographic Change in a Canadian Context*. ed. David Cheal (Toronto: University of Toronto Press, 2002), 13.

42. Jason Lian et al., "Unpaid Time Contributions by Seniors in Canada," in Independence and Economic Security in Old Age, eds. Frank T. Denton, Deborah Fretz and Byron G. Spencer (Vancouver and Toronto: UBC Press, 2000), 156.

43. Merrill Silverstein et al., "Grandparents and Grandchildren in Family Systems: A Social Development Perspective," Global Aging and Challenges to Families, eds. Vern L. Bengston and Ariel Lowenstein (New York: DeGruyter Inc., 2003), 76.

44. Lian., 174.

45. Jenny Ploeg et al., "Helping Build and Rebuild Secure Lives and Futures: Financial Transfers from Parents to Adult Children and Grandchildren," *Canadian Journal of Aging* 23, 1 (2004): S137 Table 2.

46. AARP Our first-of-its-Kind Research, <http://www.aarpfinancial.com/content/resource/gparents/gparents_research.cfm?print=y> (accessed June 25, 2008).

47. Margaret Cruikshank, *Learning to be Old: Gender, Culture and Aging* (Lanham, Boulder, New York, and Oxford: Rowman and Littlefield Publishers Inc., 2003), 182.

Chapter Six
A Woman's Best Friend is...

"Women's friendships are the connective tissue of life,"
— focus group participant

If someone asks you who your best friend is and you answer a spouse, partner, sibling, lover, mother, father, daughter, son, granddaughter/son, aunt cousin, or even yourself, of course you'd be right, it being your relationship. However, it appears that, throughout the lifecourse in many changing situations and configurations, women's best friends are other women. In fact race, ethnicity, culture, religion, health or class differences – all of which affect the way women experience life events – may not apply with respect to friendships. The importance of women's friendships seems to hold true within and across categories and cultures.

And it appears that not too much has been written until quite recently on this topic. As Sarah Greenberg and her colleagues, writing about *Friendships across the life cycle*, state "less is known . . . about the characteristics and dynamics of friendships among older women, and what role these relationships play in late life."[1] And Joanne Good – writing in the *Calgary Herald* on May 22, 2006, "That's What Girlfriends Are For" – noted that a Calgary Alberta conference in 2006 called "Circle of Friends" recognized that female friendships are too often ignored in the two-by-two world of intimate love. What was needed was talking about the qualities of friendship and the role friends play through life's ages and stages.[2] Gender is again instrumental in relation to friendships, and much has been said about the differences between women's and men's style of friendships. A couple of investigators describing these gender differences, which they acknowledge as being difficult and complex, observed that women's friendships can be seen as face-to-face and men's as side-to-side. They suggest that this could be because of differences in the socialization of women and men, the former being more inclined to establish emotionally closer relations than the latter.[3]

Where do friendships appear on mid-life boomer women's roadmaps, or given the daily hubbub of their lives, do they appear? If so what forms do they take and how central are boomer women's friendships in the new social and developmental stages of the lifecourse? One thing is pretty certain - midlife women's friendships already are and will continue to be very different than their mothers. In terms of their centrality to roadmappers, as an older boomer who is a sociologist put it "Women's friends are not just supportive to their social identity, rather, they are keystones of women's lives."⁴ The following focuses on how and why this is so is important.

Smashing Some Myths

First, to get rid of some misconceptions with respect to negative ideas about midlife and older women's friendships and aging, let's engage in a bit of myth smashing.

Myth No.1 "Most older women who are alone are isolated and depressed." Unfortunately, this is the case for some, but a large majority of women who live alone do so because they want to. A small poem attributed to Carlo Tuselli gives a nice shape to this:

> *I was dining alone*
> *Thanking myself*
> *While pouring wine*
> *Reaching for bread.*

There are many general references about unattached older women, wanting to age in place and adamant about wanting to live alone. One community research project I was involved in during the mid 1990s focusing on housing, with about sixty older female participants who all lived alone. They were unanimous in saying: "they'll have to drag me away feet first." A more recent (2006) look at single American women aged forty-five and over similarly found that far from the stereotypical view of being lonely and troubled, these women valued their independence and enjoyed being alone.[5]

Myth No.2 "It is difficult for older women to make friends later in their lives." This is simply untrue. Women in mid and later life can make new and particularly strong friendships based on mutual life experiences and common interests. In addition, the time for game-playing, envy, and competition – and the need to impress others – is long gone. Later life friendships are grounded in strength as well as in need. Of course, differences and irritations (e.g. "I'm always the one to call") exist, but are generally dealt with in a more mature fashion than is the case in one's youth. Breakups do occur, as they do in all relationships.

Myth No. 3 "Women's older years are marked by adversity and loss." Throughout the lifecourse, loss in inevitable, and more marked in late life. But what is seldom featured are the many positive aspects of later life, the existence and quality of friendships being high on the list. Many women feel that their later years provide them with the best times of their lives. Here's a representative comment: "I would never trade my amazing friends, my wonderful life for less gray hair or a flatter belly. As I've aged I've become more kind to myself and less critical of myself. I've become my own friend."[6]

From Negative to Positive

These and similar myths can cause younger and midlife women to be unnecessarily anxious about the quality of their lives in years to come and the future role of friends. For example, there is the possibility of intergenerational friendships between younger and older women. A testimonial given about the much loved Julia Child, the cooking guru who died in 2004 at the age of ninety-one, Susy Davidson, who worked with Child on *Good Morning America* referred to Child's friendship as a great gift: "She helped me redefine age, No. 1." Further, "she is the standard by which I judge all professionals. She is always eager to learn something, to try something new. She just has this generosity of spirit."[7] Another benefit of women's longer life expectancy.

Not to be overlooked is the enduring nature of women's friendships. This was a feature which drew strong responses from women in the focus groups I organized in preparation for this book. A most evocative one was the following given by a sixty-something year old: "Women's friendships are the connective tissue of life. I have always maintained my friendships. I have siblings but some aren't as important as friends, especially people you have associated with throughout your life."

And here's what another said: "I have some very long-term friends: one since I was nine years old. One who was in [nursing] training with me, and we're still very good friends." Yet another offered that she was looking forward to the arrival of a friend she'd had since Grade 2, who was coming to visit so that they could celebrate their forthcoming birthdays together. The endurance of women's friendships was expressed elsewhere, by a midlife boomer: "My longstanding friend Ruth and I have known each other since I was eight and we're now fifty-two. She provides a history for me and I for her."[8] Yet another advantage of women's friendships is that it often results in enhanced self-esteem as expressed by a woman who said: "I learned that I am valuable as a friend, that I am important to other people."[9]

Finally, the caption of a cast picture of the popular TV series *Friends*, accompanied Helen Branswell's article in the *Vancouver Sun* in June, 2005 stated that the cast of *Friends* might live longer if they stay pals. She writes "As the old saying goes, you can choose your friends but you can't choose your family. A new study suggests that if you want to live a long life, you should focus on the friends."[10] Branswell was reporting a new

Australian university study which found that there were positive survival differences among those with many friends and those with few friends: 20% of their sample who had numbers of friends outlived those with few.

Infrastructures, or, How Things are Held Together

Another familiar but older (1980s) TV series was *The Golden Girls,* quite a groundbreaker in that it dwelled on the lives, accomplishments and disappointments of four women, all previously married; three were midlife, and one in her eighties. This series, still showing in reruns, was about four women who shared living quarters as single friends. It was criticized because it seemed to be pointing to women who were "clothes horses," and mainly concerned with finding a man. However, this take overlooks the fact that, by far, these women's greatest concerns had to do with maintaining decent jobs, financial security, and health issues. Blanche, of course was depicted as highly sexual (nothing wrong with that), but it seemed clear that her greatest enjoyment came in recounting her exploits to Rose, Dorothy, and Dorothy's mother, Sophia: usually at the kitchen table, in front of a large cheesecake. The series touched on a number of situations, including job-hunting, widowhood and ageism. As Nikki

Trantner points out "They're wives, ex-wives, daughters and mothers, and as such have specific, wise views on womanhood."[11]

To move from *The Golden Girls* to the social construction of women's friendships seems to be quite a leap, but as Karen Roberto observes, relationships are at the heart and soul of women's lives, and according to her, these develop in the family. In her words "The family, where the development of personal relationships begins, provides the foundation for the formation of other informal and formal alliances."[12] She goes on to make a distinction between men's and women's friendships, noting that older women differ from older men in the way they approach and carry out exchanges between family members. As a result, women are frequently more involved with families than are men, and have greater intergenerational links than do their male counterparts.[13]

That is not to say that there aren't close friendships between women and men, far from it: "he's my best friend" is a frequent comment made about a spouse or other significant male. However, in Roberto's view, women's relationships with women friends are "often characterized as intimate and intense, words not typically used to describe friendships of older men." Other observers appear to agree, and in Ruth Harriet Jacobs words, "Close women friends are important to most women through life, and women are more self-revealing in general to their friends, than men. For many men, a wife is the confidant and friend, but many women seem to need and have relationships with women confidants."[15]

The way women approach and carry out exchanges, may, ironically, have its roots in the number of discontinuities they experience and the requirement to adjust to numerous role shifts: childbearing and childcare, changes in husband's jobs, re-entry into the labor force, widowhood, divorce, and other ruptures. It could be that the discontinuity in women's lives provides them with a basis for establishing social networks and strong social support systems. "These elements of women's lives . . . " according to Diane Gibson "have important consequences . . . women, with a lifetime of experience in maintaining and establishing social bonds with families, friendship networks, neighborhoods, voluntary associations, school associations and so forth, are simply better equipped to maintain and redevelop their social networks."[16] In other words, the interrupted nature of women's traditional lives can provide them with an environment within which they can develop and sharpen coping mechanisms which stand them in good stead to deal with the vicissitudes of life which happen in both mid and later life. Based on such experiences a woman is better able to maintain, negotiate, and renegotiate. In addition to strengthening her coping skills, she also develops more flexibility which, to use a colloquial phrase better allows her to "go with the flow." This is not, of course, to suggest that women should be grateful for adversities but, rather, that learned flexibility enables women to deal with adversities when they occur. Let's look at some of the strategies that come into play for this to happen.

Buffer Zones

It is generally recognized that women are the ones who hold families together, functioning as a kind of social glue. They are what some call 'kinkeepers'. They are the ones who maintain the family networks, organize holidays, arrange celebrations of family or friends' anniversaries and birthdays and mark religious festivals. This is the stuff of continuity, familial history and cultural traditions. The word "buffer" is occasionally used by writers and others to refer to different contexts within which women's friendships with other women play prime roles. As Jacobs sees it, discussing the general antipathy towards older women "friendships can be a buffer and a triumph of solidarity and support."[17] A buffer zone can be a kind of safety zone, a social space within which a woman can let go, talk of the compromises she may make in her daily life which she may resent and which angers her. Such buffer zones are provided by friendships with other women, within which she can find self-validation through shared experiences. It is not possible to overestimate the importance of being able to express one's feelings within a relatively relaxed environment. How many times have we heard other women say "I thought I was the only one who felt like this?"

And, just as important or perhaps even more important, women's get togethers can be a lot of fun – what some refer to as being "gal pals." Ellen Goodman and Patricia O'Brien, writing in *I Know Just What You Mean: The Power of Friendship in Women's Lives*, have a very upbeat take on this. They discuss the ways they (the co-authors) talked and talked and talked for over a quarter of a century "and in that time we had become fluent in the language of female friendship."[18] This idea of a language of friendship is intriguing. It sheds some light on aspects of women's friendships that are intangible, and hard to express, but are active ingredients in friendships nevertheless. They go on to say "So on we go, laughing, complaining, playing, poking fun, having fun. The fun that exists both in the moment and in the memory, feeling known and understood, the whole elusive thing."[19] There is no doubt as to the capacity of women to have fun. If you have ever been in a restaurant where a group of office staff women is celebrating somebody's birthday, their laughter can be heard across the room, to put it mildly. As reported in the *Edmonton Journal*, February 27,

2008, one woman reluctant to join a group said, "As soon as I started hanging out with gals, I realized that it was healthy for me . . . like every female experience, it's going out with your friends and laughing and eating." When I went to see Helen Mirren in *The Queen,* I saw a small group of women in the line-up, each of whom was wearing a gold foil crown, laughing up a storm. Single women are traveling together a great deal, in fact there is one travel agency which organizes tours for menopausal women, certainly a recognition of more loose attitudes among today's mid-life women. I cannot imagine such a thing even being dreamed of in my generation. I also heard from a group of four midlife women who have been friends since high school, going away together to celebrate their fiftieth birthday year. There are also many midlife women exercise and fitness buffs, who both run and attend fitness classes together.

Married women's friendships also provide them with buffer zones. Marriage simply cannot provide a woman with all of her personal and social needs. As O'Connor explains "The acceptable role for women's friendships in this scenario is complementing the marital relationship, that is, providing practical and emotional resources which, for various reasons, are not or cannot be provided by the marital relationship."[20] Often, a husband or partner may feel uncomfortable or even threatened by his wife's closeness with her female friends, a situation that may result in certain constraints, such as the wife limiting the number of times she goes out with her friends. There are a number of things that married and partnered women feel they can only talk about to close women friends. These things may include finances or sexuality. With reference to her intimate friend, one woman commented: "She is good to talk things over with. It's only Brenda really that I discuss my worries with."[21] Another women declares "Beatrice feels she cannot talk to her husband about the awful time she is going through . . . 'he knows my anxieties and fears.' When asked if he was able to help her, she replied 'No, not one bit. Not one bit .He just doesn't understand. He can't.'"[22] Though in the context of marriage or partnerships, these anecdotes again suggest the language of women's friendships.

I end this section with a quote from Terri Apter and Ruthellen Jesselson's study. They offer the thoughts of one of their interviewees regarding the ability of women to sustain lifelong friendships. "These women also came to value the shared experiences, the long-term knowledge that they had of each other. When asked what had kept her in contact with her best friend of thirty years, Dorothy grinned and said, "Alyssa is the only person in the world who has known all my husbands and all my lovers – and seen every apartment or house I've ever lived in. Alyssa is my continuity in life. Men come and men go. My children think I was born when they were. Alyssa is the record of my life, and I am the same to her." And she adds: "to a lifelong friend, you don't have to explain much of anything about yourself."[23] Quite a testimony to the centrality of friendships in women's lives.

Mother/Daughter Bonds

Although this topic could be a part of the Buffer Zone section, it is a topic much on the minds of both midlife and older women. Discussions often emphasize that mother/daughter relations are either reviled or revered of the "I couldn't do without her" type or the "We don't get along" variety. It is a touchy subject, because these bonds occur differently in different situations. And in addition, it is often the case that a mother/daughter bond, where there are several female siblings, may exist more strongly with one particular daughter than the others.

I turn now to a small, community based study conducted by Rosemary Bliezner and colleagues *Diversity and Dynamics in Late-Life Mother-Daughter Relationships*[24] and I take late-life to mean beyond the contexts of teens, sibling rivalries, and young adults, and more likely mid-life women and their mothers. This American study aimed to get some qualitative information based on women's experiences, expressed in the words of the participants. All of the following short sections are taken from that study. The investigators looked at three major aspects of the mother-daughter relationships: (1) companionship (2) cohesion (i.e. feelings of closeness and togetherness; and (3) conflict that is the extent of and reactions to disagreements. Here are some of the things the women said.

Companionship

One mother commented: "I don't know what I'd do without her . . . We shop together and work some in the yard together. Since I lost my husband, I don't know if I give as much to her as she gives to me." Another woman said, "She's always willing to do what she can, [for example] give me advice about a doctor . . . [We] help her out 'cause she was left alone with four boys." And another ["My daughter] is all I have . . . I think we go very well together. I couldn't do without her, and I don't think she could do without me." Bliezner et al. found two patterns – one in which the mothers gave more than they received, the other in which the exchanges were more balanced exchanges with more reciprocity.

Several mothers felt that open communication enables feelings of closeness between them and their daughters: "She tells a person how she feels. She don't beat around the bush"; "I talk to her two or three times a day. If she's too busy during the call she always calls me at night"; and "I love to hear her opinions, so she'll give me her opinions. Then she'll say 'now you have to think that over for yourself, Mother.'" In difficult relationships, communication is less frequent and less beneficial: "We don't share much together. I don't tell her nothing. We don't discuss feelings." The analysts felt that many mothers and daughters enjoyed and valued each other's company, although difficulties could cause tensions.

Cohesion

In the study, one woman said: "We go for lunch. We go shopping . . . I may go three or four days a week and not see her, but we talk."; another "I was telling [my daughter] that I would rather go in a nursing home than to bother them. She said not as long as she lived . . . So, you couldn't ask for nothing more than that I wouldn't think," and this: "She helped me out with my problems. If things don't go right, she stands by her mother." And still another: "She's very thoughtful. She thinks about us [if] she goes away . . .they always call. We know where they are. She's just very thoughtful." Here, the authors note there is a sense of importance to mothers of feeling close to their daughters and they clearly value that feeling.

Conflict

Bliezner et al. found that some mothers denied that they had any disagreements, while others claimed they never argued. Only a few of the mothers indicated extensive conflict, usually within the context of the daughter's problems. From one who reported no conflicts: "I can reason with [daughter] and she understands. We never have an argument. Not that we're perfect, but it's just not necessary." Another noted, "A lot of people, if they can find the least little thing, they just build it up and up. But we don't do that."

A daughter in the study commented: "We don't disagree very much. I don't bother . . . she's an old lady now and knows her own business. I don't interfere at all. If we ever disagree about things, I just keep it to myself." The woman who seemed to have the most serious conflict with her daughter commented: "She always has been a big problem to us . . . it's usually about neglecting her children. Rarely will she tell me the truth and tell me if anything is wrong."

The authors conclude, in part, that close mother-daughter relationships in adulthood are likely to include satisfying interactions, a history that displays little conflict, involve few control issues, and have many opportunities for informal contact. It also seems that some of the conflicts reported are carry-overs from mother-daughter incompatibility in earlier years.

While the study is small, and not generalizable, it recognizes the strength of adult mother-daughter friendships and some noted difficulties. Certainly from my own experience, my relationship with my mother was such that I did not confide many things, mainly because she was quite a bit older than I was, and also came from a different culture. I can say that my friendships with my boomer daughters is of critical importance to me, even though we certainly have occasional differences, we are close.

These few examples are mere indication of the complexities inherent in the mother/daughter bond.

Shock Absorbers

The idea of shock absorbers is intended to indicate the emotional intensity of women's friendships, especially those who face critical times. When they have to deal with some of life's most demanding situations, women are helped immensely by their friendships with other women. I asked several of my midlife friends to write down the times in their lives when their female friends helped them the most. Here are several of their statements:

• "When my friend Lisa was very sick with kidney failure, and had been in and out of the hospital, her partner who had been her primary care provider was called out of town to deal with one of his parent's rapidly deteriorating health. Darlene, one of Lisa's friends, organized care through a network of her friends. She made a list of Lisa's friends, called them all and coordinated their visits and stays with Lisa over several weeks. People brought food, or spent the night, or did a "day shift." In this way, Lisa always had someone with her, in case she needed immediate medical attention. It was terrific. Darlene's organization made you feel not only that you were helping Lisa, but also that you were part of a "community," that you were connected through Lisa to a wide network of friends."

- When my husband of many years had an affair and wanted to leave me and our children, who were still at home, I was distraught. I truly believe I could never have endured the emotional trauma I experienced without the love, support and guidance I received from two very close women friends: an older-and-wiser-than-me female co-worker, and a gutsy sister-in-law. Day after day, while the crisis unfolded, my friends were there for me: on the phone early and late; serving me endless cups of coffee in their kitchens while drying my tears; bolstering my self-esteem and offering sage advice;

using their friendship with my husband to remind him of what he would be losing. A sister-in-law called him a "dumb dodo" and urged him to "get over this foolishness" before he alienated both sides of the family. Fortunately, the affair proved to be relatively short-lived. Our marriage survived, and in some ways was improved thanks in part to the wise input of my wonderful women friends."

- "My bosom buddy [name] and I have been "there" for each other, going through breast cancer not once but twice – different details and treatments, but very similar feelings, ranging from utter confusion and despair to insight and hope, helping each other to find meaning in this "journey". (I joke that we have a poor travel agent – taking this journey once was enough, we didn't need to repeat it.) Anyway, our shared experience has allowed us more candour than has been possible with any other relationships and that is a blessing."

- [speaking of the death of her mother] "The fact that these women gave me unconditional caring really helped me through this difficult period. I think that one thing women can do is "be there" for you in many different ways. There is a kind of eloquence that exists between women friends, who can hug you just when you need it and nothing else needs to be said."

- "A friend, Margaret who is in her eighties, was hit by a car in a crosswalk as she and her sister, also in her eighties, were crossing the street on a dark, rainy night. She suffered not only smashed bones which threatened to cost her a foot, but in addition, her beloved sister succumbed to her injuries. Margaret was in the hospital for months enduring operations to save her foot, and during this awful time, a friend of hers named Jean who lived next door and had a key to the house, went to Margaret's computer and found her e-mail addresses. Jean then wrote to Margaret's whole friendship network, informing us all that she was taking the role of communicator so that none of us had to be in the dark about what was happening. Throughout the months of Margaret's hospital stay, Jean issued regular bulletins about her condition, letting us know that Margaret's spirits were lifted by our letters, cards, and gifts. Thankfully, her foot was saved."

These abbreviated case histories, the personal memoirs of the help given by their women friends in times of dire need, demonstrate the extraordinary nature of women's friendships. Such examples of women being shock absorbers could no doubt be replicated myriad times. One of the most crucial times for women's friendships comes when women lose a partner.

Widowhood – Not Always but Occasionally Merry

One of life's most shattering events is the loss of a spouse or partner. This is always a shock. Perhaps if the loved one has suffered a prolonged illness, the death may be a relief. Much has been written in Canada and elsewhere about the hazards of widowhood, including the loss not only of status, but a downward slide of income. As Chappell et al. indicate: "One of the most striking characteristics of elderly widows is their straitened economic circumstances; approximately one-half of Canadian elder widows live in poverty."[25]

We also know that women are more likely to be widowed in later life than are men and to live longer either alone or with family, while men are more likely to remarry after the death of a spouse. By the time a woman reaches the age of seventy-five, there is a strong likelihood that she will be widowed. Hopefully, given better health practices and medical advances, widowhood may occur later in midlife women's lives. But it will still likely be a stumbling block for boomer roadmaps, in addition to its occurrence in the lives of their parents.

Widowhood is not just an event; rather, it is a transition that takes place over time and involves various stages of grief and depression. At the end of the acute grieving period, which may last a year or more, the widow must then go through reengagement. At this time widows may begin to look forward to involvement with social relations.

This period may include previous friends or new ones, as the woman transforms herself from being half of a couple to being single, not an easy thing to do. One of the older women, a widow in one of the focus groups I conducted, said that although for years she and her husband had been part of a couple's group – going to dinner, playing cards and traveling together – she was dropped by most of these couples when she became widowed. One would think that in this modern age, with all the changes to family dynamics, including rising numbers of single women, such anachronistic behavior would no longer exist. However, this does not appear to be the case. Another widowed focus group woman noted rather sardonically "I don't get invited to dinners anymore, but only to lunch. Maybe the other wives don't like odd numbers at their tables, or maybe they think their husband has a roving eye." And one of the women put it thus "but you don't come to a couples' dance as a single person because you won't feel welcome. I think the wives think we are a threat."

Another possible take was described in this way: "As well, when a husband dies, a widow is dropped like a hot potato from the girlfriend network . . . I think because it's a discomfort for others when seeing them as not part of a couple."[26] This suggests that some of widow's associates don't want to be reminded of their own vulnerability. Apparently maintaining friendships with couples remains difficult for a single woman living in couples-oriented society. There seems to be a cultural lag in that many people haven't recognized that so many more women are single today than was the case a few decades ago.

Happily, the above examples of widowhood exclusion are far from being the whole picture, because in the nature of women's friendships, neighbors, friends, and families are the "connective tissue" that help to overcome the disjuncture of widowhood helping women to cope with loss. A support network can play a critical role immediately following the loss and later during the re-engagement phase. Laura Hurd, who wrote *WE'RE NOT OLD!*, observes that "friendships with other women play a vital role in a woman's reconstruction of her identity as a widowed, single, older person."[29]

A significant amount of time was spent on the topic of widowhood and friendships by focus group participants. Their comments are particularly insightful. Here are some: "My friends helped me – my hiking pals and my mates at the Police Department where I volunteer." Another noted, "My buddies at work helped me" and another woman noted "My bridge group has been there to this day – a wonderful support – we were a support group all through the years from the time our children were in school. Whenever we had problems, we'd take them to the bridge club." One woman commented on a friend who was not quite so helpful: "I had a really good friend – now she's dating my son." It seems that many different scenarios play themselves out when one loses a spouse.

The positive skills that stand midlife and older women in good stead generally, the ability to give and receive support, also apply when they face widowhood. Consequent upon a period of grieving, many women begin to recognize certain gains in their lives. Not many widows will mark their widowhood(s) as did Catharina Ustings Ras, a seventeenth-century vintner who, upon losing five husbands, developed a wine blended from five different grape varieties in order to honour them.[28] It is to be hoped that contemporary widows will not have the misfortune of losing so many husbands (never mind finding them in the first place), but many widows do mark their new status in ways that become important strengths to them. For example, while most widows feel the loss of their husband and their role as wife very intensely, as Chappell et al note for some the experience of widowhood can be what they term "an ambiguous loss."[29] In other words, losing a bad spouse can be a relief and a blessing in disguise. Given that the older generation of women leaned more towards staying in an unhappy marriage than in leaving it, "future cohorts of widows will be less likely to face the challenge of having to appear bereaved when they are actually glad, or at least, relieved that their husband is dead."[30] Perhaps we are too timid, or feel it politically incorrect to mark a number of positive things about widowhood, but like many other changes in status, they create opportunities for growth and development.

It seems there had been a shift from a "gloom and doom" portrayal of widowhood to a portrayal that emphasizes strength, interpersonal skills, and personal development. For example, a positive aspect of widowhood is the opportunity it offers to present a new identity: one different than that based on being a wife or partnered person. A newly single woman, given time, can become engaged in activities, not as one-half of a couple but, rather, as wholly herself. If she is in the paid workforce, she may relate differently to her female co-workers, perhaps joining them for a' girl's night out.' A most encouraging achievement of post-widowhood especially for women who do not wish to remarry or enter into another relationship is that of a new independence. This is what psychologists used to refer to as an "aha!" experience – a sudden insight or recognition. Widowhood may offer a woman new ways of being in the world, sometime expressed as "saying no feels good," a reference to the times partnered women make compromises that are not in their interests or against their wishes.

The focus group women went to town on this one. Here is a collection of some of their remarks about their experiences as widows:

- "People ask me why I am not married. I sure wouldn't want to be married to anyone like the men my friends are married to."

- Another felt that "Once older women find their independence, they keep on and they are not afraid to voice their opinions. They stop saying 'my husband says.'"

- "I've turned into a beast: I don't take crap from anyone. I am outspoken.

- "My husband used to do all the finances, but I've learned to do this and can handle it myself now. "

- "I've cooked my last meal – I eat what I want, when I want."

• "At last I have control of the [TV] clicker."

• "He was boring."

These comments may be seen as trivial, but they are the expressions of a group of everyday women's responses to real life situations. The issue is that within the context of a woman being released from what may have been a restricted context, these statements can be seen as evidence of new-found control and independence.

Their freedom in expressing such feelings also attests to the safe environment they were in – a group of supportive peers, who formed a buffer zone. It seems that numbers of older women are engaging in the 'grey divorce', as noted in the previous chapter, thus probably avoiding widowhood.

Older Lesbians and Friendship

Friendships among older lesbians are not something the heterosexual world knows a great deal about. The Canadian analyst Ingrid Connidis sums it up well. "At the moment, the tendency to ignore same-sex partnerships makes it necessary to give these relationships special attention, both because there is less known about them and because we must emphasize the importance of including them."[31]

Long-term relationships between lesbians may be more common than is usually assumed. Karen Roberto helps to understand in what ways lesbian friendships differ from straight ones. "Older lesbians involved in long-term committed relationships generally provide each other with a comprehensive, mutual support system and the economic advantages of sharing homes and resources."[32]

She goes on to explain lesbian relationships are similar to heterosexual ones in that they provide emotional, tangible support, along with nurturance and acceptance. However "Despite their mutual commitment, the political and prejudicial realities of the world in which they live often prohibit lesbians from openly acknowledging the nature of their relationship."[33] When a lesbian loses a partner, her transition may well be more difficult than it is for heterosexual women.

Mary Hunt, a feminist theologian, has written a powerful analysis of women and gays living in a culturally-restricted world. Discussing the difficulties lesbians experience in a male-dominated world, and the consequent fear of making same-sex alliances public, Hunt states: "This has led many women to shy away from identifying their friendships with women, even those that include no explicit genital sexual expression, for fear of suffering from the stigma of homosexuality in a homophobic culture."[34]

Like heterosexual relationships, gay and lesbian relationships are diverse. Consider the following engaging dialog between fifty-plus year old gays and lesbians who were interviewed by *50 Plus Online Magazine* in December 2004:

Interviewer: How do gay and lesbian seniors fit in with the rest of society?

Larry: It depends on where you live, what kind of job you have . . . the degree to which gays and lesbians are "out" can vary. Older homosexuals are far less secure about their sexuality than those who are younger. It wasn't as if the doors swung open and all of us danced out.

Ellen: the youth-oriented culture is often associated with gay and lesbian communities, [and this] can have the unfortunate effect of isolating seniors.

Ruth: Often, closeted seniors live alone or with partners without any additional support. I know many of us feel that younger gays and lesbians who are in their 40s and 50s, you know, just a little behind us, should reach out and take on more responsibility . . .

Edward: There are many downsides to getting old but there are plenty of rewards.[35]

Sound familiar?

Diversity among lesbians and gays, apart from the schism between older and younger ones alluded to in the above interview, includes the degree to which their families and other associates are accepting and supportive. A family's non-acceptance of same sex partnerships clearly puts additional strains on these relationships.

Nonetheless, straight women can learn much from lesbians, not the least of which is how to weather transitions during which they face additional strains. As Suzanne Slater, writing *The Lesbian Family Life Cycle*, notes: "The nature of the couple's emotional and physical intimacy may likewise be affected as they enter a stage of life containing difficult compromises and likely personal losses."[36] Also, it is unlikely that the division of labor in a same-sex household will be as lopsided as it is in heterosexual households, even among dual career partners. In fact this may present straight women with a model of equity. It also seems that lesbians continue to be close following break-ups, which may have something to do with the closeness that often develops between members of an oppressed minority. Slater tells us of one older lesbian who noted: "Nina and her lover Ellen went to visit their neighbor, Jan, who had recently been widowed. 'You two are so lucky,' Jan told the couple, 'You may still have each other for years to come . . .' The irony of the conversation struck Nina at that moment. Her mother had been so afraid that without a husband, Nina would grow old alone. Now, here was this heterosexual friend envying Nina's greater chance of being partnered through the rest of her life."[37]

Case History

Marion is a lesbian in her late fifties, a professional who occupies a top post in the institution at which she works. She recognized that she had feelings for other women when she was about nineteen, when she became attracted to her female sports coach. Nevertheless, she entered a traditional heterosexual marriage, during which time two sons were born. Towards the eighteenth year of this marriage, her lesbian feelings became prominent. She and her husband discussed it, and agreed that, for the sake of the boys, they should stay together until the oldest one was fifteen and in high school.

Her parents each reacted differently to the news that Marion was a lesbian and leaving her heterosexual marriage. Her father, a physician of a liberal bent, was understanding, but her mother, who believed in traditional marriage, was angry. During one family dinner Marion's mother threw the main course, a stew, into the garbage pail. Marion's sons were also very angry, the older boy deflecting his feelings by focusing on sports. Although he is not gay, he came to know boys who were, and this gave him a sense that there were many people other than his mother who were engaged in same-sex relationships. He felt abandoned and refused to talk to her for two years. The younger boy took his anger out on his older brother. "These were pretty hard times," Marion reflects. Fortunately, she had a sister who was supportive. The divorce came after a planned separation, with Marion and her husband attending counseling and mediation. She also went to see a psychiatrist, who said she should be more like her mother and learn to like ironing, polishing silver, and cooking, which made her ask herself: "What the hell am I doing here?"

Marion considers herself "out" in that her close friends at work know that she is a lesbian; however, she has overheard others in the organization in which she works make derogatory remarks about her.

She is not in a relationship at present. She was in a relationship with another woman for a number of years, but her partner left to go and live with a man. They are still close. And now that her mother is older and more accepting, the four of them go out occasionally – Marion, her mother, her former partner, and the latter's new partner. One of her more recent partners displayed jealousy of Marion's strong attachment to her mother, and Marion left the relationship because of this.

Now as a midlife woman, Marion recognized that her marriage was an emotional void. When she was in her twenties and thirties, her desire for intimacy with other women was confusing. She had to find her inner self in relation to her sexuality. She feels differently now: sex is not nearly as important to her as it once was. She now feels she could relate to the kind of intimacy that offers holding, cuddling, and back rubs. She is content with her life now. Her mother, now ailing, has moved in with her. They have separate quarters but eat or watch TV together if they feel like it. Marion believes that lesbianism and heterosexuality are blurred, that they do not have clear boundaries. Although she is happy alone, she would not reject a compatible relationship.[38] This is only one example of what is no doubt a range of different experiences of friendship among midlife lesbian women – we need to learn more from and about them.

Sisterhood is Powerful

Considerable attention is currently being paid to the relationship between sisters as they grow older. Previously, interest focused upon childhood experiences, and in particular, sibling rivalry. Discussing the topic of supportive sisters, Karen Roberto has this to say: "Sibling ties in later life exist within a myriad of contexts . . . and the larger family

342

system. It is perhaps the longest kin relationship of older women. The sibling relationship is built upon a shared family history that provides a basis for mutual emotional support and understanding. Ties with siblings seem to wane sometime during the first part of adulthood, but resume after preoccupations with the procreative family subside."[39] On the question of closeness between sisters, or sister pairs, it appears that there is more closeness and friendship between sisters than between brothers or between brothers and sisters. This is a broad overview and of course sisters and brothers are certainly friends, but according to Terri Apter, writing in *The Sister Knot: Why we fight, why we're jealous, and why we'll love each other no matter what* (a title which seems to pretty well say it all), "Sisters more than brothers support each other through the major tasks and events of adulthood: marriage, childrearing, divorce, widowhood, aging and dying."[40] It does appear that there is more closeness between sisters than between brothers.

What follows is a brief glimpse of the work of Ingrid Connidis, an acknowledged Canadian expert on siblings. In her opinion, the place of adult siblings has received very limited research attention, despite what she considers to be a unique feature of the sibling relationship – that of its duration. The sibling relationship offers the potential for shared experiences over a lifetime, providing a ready basis for reminiscence as we age. Sibling relationships clearly provide a sense of continuity over the lifecourse. Eighty percent of people aged sixty-five and or more have at least one living sibling. According to Connidis: "This will be even more true of the baby boom generation, whose older members are now in middle age. Most of us can expect to have at least one surviving brother or sister well into old age."[41]

Siblings will play an important role on midlife boomer's roadmaps as they grow older. The growing complexities of family life, given the prevalence of divorce and remarriage means that in the future more adults will have both half- and step-siblings, family situations which are already part of some boomers' family experience.

Connidis points out that geographical proximity tends to have an important impact on sibling interaction. She cites a seventy-year-old brother discussing his relationship with his younger sister upon retiring. "Oh, it hasn't changed any. Still have the geographic distance . . . but it really doesn't matter because the telephone's a wonderful instrument, and she knows and I know that if either of us needs the other, we're on the next plane."[42] With regard to companionship and intimacy, those who are widowed, single, or childless are closer to their siblings than are married partners: "The high rate of widowhood among older people makes siblings pivotal or focal kin for many in old age, particularly women."[43] Further, compared to men, middle-aged and older women report being closer to their siblings regardless of gender. In a study of persons aged sixty-five and older, Connidis found that 22% listed a sibling as one of their key confidants.

Later in life, the close proximity of sisters in childhood may be recreated. Women, as we well know, tend to outlive their male partners by several years, and many widowed and retired sisters end up living again in the same kind of intimacy as they shared in childhood. As Connidis expresses it, at the end of her life, as at the beginning, a sister may be privy to the small, personal details about the other . . . to which possibly no other person except a long-term sexual partner ever has access. Over a whole lifetime, such intimacy contributes to a rare and special kind of closeness.[44]

Not all sister relations are of the Pollyanna variety. The issue of competitiveness and rivalry is examined by Terri Apter, sometimes starting in childhood as sibling rivalry and can carry on, with scenarios playing and replaying over the lifecourse. She cites well-known rivalries which existed between a couple of famous sisters, Ann Landers and Abigail Van Buren, who were twins, "each raced to whatever goal the other set her sights on . . . " There was also the De Havilland sisters of movie fame, Olivia and Joan Fontaine. According to

Apter, they remained frozen in competition, to a point where Olivia refused to accept her first Oscar . . . when she learned that Joan would be presenting it.[45] The question of competitiveness may also be evident when it comes to parents who are failing. A study of adult siblings Apter notes, found half the families reporting conflict over care-giving arrangements, and can even persist after a parent's death. She does say however "The shared world of siblings has a lifelong power. So closely bound is one sister to another that it may never by possible to dissociate oneself psychologically from one's sibling . . . in a sibling, we see how closely our pasts hug themselves to our present lives."[46]

And, finally and unavoidably, the downside to older women's friendship bonds is the loss of friends in later life. Facing the loss of friends is intense for older women and men, constantly reminding them of their own mortality and thinning ranks. My late, dear friend Lanie Melamed, whom I met in my (our) seventies, both of us having so much in common in our likes and dislikes, died a few short years ago of breast cancer despite fighting tooth and nail to beat it. It left a big hole in my life and I miss her to this very day. Such losses invoke deep grief. Some turn to religion for comfort, some turn to family, some to partners, some to their remaining friends. Others turn to yoga, meditation or other personal sources of strength. The current pop psychology about "bringing closure" after a loss fails to recognize that, when we lose someone we loved truly, madly, deeply, there is never "closure." A remembered event, scenario, or anniversary, a birthday or Christmas causes many a lump in the throat years after the loss has occurred. "Closure" is perhaps applicable to those seeking justice through the courts. It is not applicable to those who have lost someone they loved with a passion. Of course, it need hardly be said that someone suffering severe, prolonged depression and unable to move forward should consult a professional mental health expert, or a community-based mental health group if one is available.

We now have convincing evidence of the reciprocity and rewards women receive through their friendships in a variety of situations. But, if further convincing is required, there appears to be scientific evidence which strengthens this premise. In a study on stress by the University of California in Los Angeles, the researchers found that in contrast to the male 'flight or fight syndrome', women react to stress with a more 'tend and befriend' response. The difference in the response may be because the hormone oxytocin is released in women, which produces a calming effect, and this release evidently does not occur in men. The researchers find further that other studies on human males and females show that underlying conditions of stress, the desire to affiliate with others is substantially more marked among females than males. Additionally, in relation to social networks, women are more likely [30%] than men to have provided some type of support, including economic, work-related difficulties, interpersonal problems, death and negative health events.

They do not suggest that men do not perform such activities but question why most stress research has been on male behavior.[47] Whether or not this study stands up after future testing remains to be seen. It is an intriguing approach, and may provide a scientific basis to the importance of women's friendships. If, indeed, such 'proof' is needed.

Boomer women's friendships are hugely different than those of the women in previous generations. Unlike their parents, boomers grew up in a loose, wired, fast-moving technological world; went to rock concerts *en masse*; spent a lot of time getting an education; were exposed to a variety of lifestyles and living arrangements, including communes. In the 60s and 70s the women's movement stressed egalitarianism, friendships were voluntary, as most are, and strived to be rid of power ploys. Rebecca Adams and Rosemary Blieszner think "a hallmark of the baby boomers when they were young adults was a feeling of freedom to acknowledge emotions and express them more directly to more types of people than had been done before. Openness and honesty were goals for friendship and other close relations." Women in the older generation rarely, if ever, discussed sex or finances, for example.

Given that the majority of boomer women are in the labor force and multi-tasking, there is little time for relaxed lunches, bridge games, or community get-togethers on midlife women's roadmaps. They may not find the same time as did their mothers to invest in developing friendships. Still, the prevalence of cell phones, text messaging, and e-mail provides ways for women in the fast-forward lanes to continue to communicate with friends.

One older boomer woman I spoke to on this topic told me she and long-time girlfriends, all in the workforce now, meet on a set night once a month, calling themselves "the bridge club," although the get-togethers have nothing to do with bridge.

It is unlikely that boomer women will stay in unhappy marriages, as is evidenced by high divorce rates. Their work association will likely provide them with a rich source of camaraderie in addition to their lifelong association with family and friends. The importance of female bonding has existed through the ages and across cultures. As boomer women proceed on their roadmap continuing to shape new social stages and new behavioral friendship patterns, these are and will continue to be vastly different than those of previous generations. But it is hard to think that friendships with other women will be any less important than they have ever been.

Things You Can Do As A Boomer Woman Change Agent:

• If a close friend loses her spouse or partner, you might enquire about a spousal bereavement group in your community, from which you feel she could benefit. Or perhaps starting one yourself if there are none.

• If a friend is enduring an acrimonious divorce, or is recently widowed, urge her to get out and try forming a new identity when she is open to this, by doing something she never did with her partner so there are no memories. Perhaps by joining a group, for e.g. starting fitness classes, going ice-skating or joining a walking group: women's walking groups are quite common as are investment groups. There is a lot on the internet about midlife singles.

• Confront anyone who refers to women's get-togethers as "bitching" or "gossiping" sessions. There is the classic anecdote about a man approaching a table in a restaurant where two women are dining, and asking "Are you alone?" Make sure they understand the strong and self-reliant nature of women's friendships and networks.

- There are times when good friends may not be as available as they usually are. A mid-life woman who is taking further training, or going back to school, or caring for a needful parent is more limited in the time she can spend. This requires recognition of her changed situation, and not resentment because she has less time.

- There are women who have many friends, and others who have few. Having few friends does not mean a deficiency of any kind. There are some for whom one close, good friend is sufficient and mutually satisfying.

References

1. Sarah Greenberg et al., "Friendship Across the Life Cycle: A Support Group for Older Women," *Journal of Gerontological Social Work* 32, 4 (1999): 8.

2. <http://www.canada.com/topics/lifestyle.relationships/story.html?id_3feb7360-5c00-4d20-9.> (accessed August 11, 2006).

3. Rebecca G. Adams, Rosemary Bleiszner, and Brian DeVries, "The Definitions of Friendship in the Third Age: Age, Gender and Study Location Effects," *Journal of Aging Studies* 14, 1 (2000): 3.

4. Melody Hessing, Sociologist, personal communication, March 2005.

5. Sarah Mahoney, "The Secret Lives of Single Women," May & June, 2006, <http://www.aarpmagazine.org/lifestyle/single_women.html.> (accessed March 13, 2007).

6. Gerry Hurwitz, e-mail message to author, February 13, 2005.

7. Associated Press, *Globe and Mail*, August 14, 2004, R3.

8. Cited by Joanne Good, "That's What Girlfriends are for," *Calgary Herald*, May 22, 2006.

9. Nan Stevens, "Combatting Loneliness: A Friendship Enrichment Programme for Older Women," *Aging and Society* 21, 2 (2001): 193.

10. Helen Brandswell, "Close Friends Help Elderly Live Longer, Study Finds," *Vancouver Sun*. June 16, 2005.

11. Nikki Trantner, *The Golden Girls: The Complete First Season*, November 23, 2004, <http://www.popmatters.com/tv.previews.g/golden-girls-season-1-dvd.shtml> (accessed March 1, 2005).

12. Karen A. Roberto, "Older Women's Relationships: Weaving Lives Together," in *Women as They Age*, ed. J. Dianne Garner and Susan O. Mercer (Birmingham and New York: Howarth Press, 2001), 115.

13. Ibid.

14. Ibid.

15. Ruth Harriet Jacobs, "Friendships among Old Women," *Journal of Women and Aging*, 2, 2 (1990): 20-21.

16. Diane Gibson, "Broken Down by Age and Gender: The Problem of Older Women," *Gender and Society* 10, 4 (1996): 422.

17. Jacobs, "Friendships," 28.

18. Ellen Goodman and Patricia O'Brien, *I Know Just What You Mean: The Power of Friendships in Women's Lives* (New York: Simon & Schuster, 2000): 12.

19. Ibid., 103 (emphasis the authors').

20. Pat O'Connor, *Friendship Between Women: A Critical Review* (New York: Harvester Wheatsheaf, 1992), 56.

21. Ibid., 63.

22. Frida Furman, *Facing the Mirror: Older Women and Beauty Shop Culture* (New York and London: Routledge, 1997): 32.

23. Terri Apter and Ruthellen Jesselson, *Best Friends: The Pleasures and Perils of Girls' and Women's Friendships* (New York: Crown Publishers, 1998), 279-80.

24. Rosemary Bliezner et al, "Diversity and Dynamics in Late-Life Mother-Daughter Relationships," *Journal of Women and Aging* 8, 34 (1996): 5-24.

25. Neena Chappell et al., *Aging in Contemporary Canada* (Toronto: Prentice Hall, 2003), 300.

26. Good, "That's what Girlfriends are for," op.cit.

27. Laura C. Hurd, "WE'RE NOT OLD! Older Women's Negotiations of Aging and Oldness," *Journal of Aging Studies* 13, 4 (Toronto: Prentice Hall, 2001): 422.

28. *Vancouver Sun*, March 5, 2005.

29. Cited in Chappell et al., *Aging*, 301.

30. Ibid.

31. Ingrid Arnett Connidis, *Family Ties and Aging* (Thousand Oaks: Sage Publications, 2001), 60.

32. Roberto, "Older Women's Relationships," 117.

33. Ibid.

34. Mary E. Hunt, *Fierce Tenderness: A Feminist Theology of Friendships*. (New York: Crossroads, 1991), 43.

35. Garry Geyer, "Being Gay or Lesbian and Past 50," 50 Plus Magazine, <http://www.50plusmag.com/

50plusissues/1201004gaylesbian/120104gaylesbian.html>
(accessed December 17, 2005).

36. Suzanne Slater, *The Lesbian Family Life Cycle* (New York: Free Press, 1995), 221.

37. Ibid.211.

38. Personal communication, March 2004. The respondent wishes to remain anonymous. Marion is not her real name.

39. Roberto, "Older Women's Relationships," 121.

40. Terri Apter, *The Sister Knot*: Why we fight, Why we're jealous and Why we'll love each other no matter what. New York, London: Norton. (2007). 269.

41. Connidis, *Family Ties*, 209.

42. Ibid., 210.

43. Ibid., 219.

44. Ibid., 220. passim.

45. Apter, op.cit., 263-264.

46. Ibid., 262.

47. S.E.Klein et al "Female Response to Stress: Tend and Befriend," *Psychological Review* 107, 3 (2000): 411-429.

48. Rebecca G. Adams and Rosemary Blieszner, "Baby Boomer Friendships" *Generations: Journal of the American Society on Aging* 22, 1 (1998): 74.

Chapter Seven

From Raging Hormones
to Raging Grannies

Some say the world will end in fire
Some in ice
From what I've tasted of desire
I hold with those who favour fire ...
    — *Robert Frost*

"Life should NOT be journey to the grave with the intention of arriving safely in an attractive and well preserved body, but rather to skid in sideways, chocolate in one hand, wine in the other, body thoroughly used up, totally worn out and screaming 'Woo Hoo what a ride.'" This tongue-in-cheek advice is often circulated via e-mails or as posters by pundits on International Women's Day, which they rename "Very Good Looking and Damn Smart Women's Day."

A 2004 obituary which ran in the *Vancouver Sun* had this heading "Our Mother Wore Purple." It went on to say that their mother had worn purple clothes and a red hat, spending her money on chocolates, summer gloves, and satin sandals. She sat down on the pavement when tired, gobbled samples in shops, and served her guests flaming gin-soaked raisins. Clearly this woman's children were expressing their admiration for a mother who flaunted rules of appropriate behavior, doing things "her way".

While most mid-life women might prefer to reach their later years in a less flamboyant fashion, they will likely face a number of issues on their roadmaps taking a more sober and innovative approach if they are to achieve a secure future, both culturally and economically. In the Prologue to this book I outlined three themes: (1) women's increased longevity creating a new historical stage of the life cycle, (2) the developmental possibilities inherent within this stage, and (3) the importance of popular culture in influencing the negative images many women have of themselves, and the way they come to view their aging. I also noted that boomers are far from homogeneous, that they differ from each other in terms of their ages and stages, which present a number of contradictions in their lifecourses. The three themes informed the topics which this book addressed: persistent ageism and the iconic image of youth; cultural aspects of aging different than biological aging; health issues and the recognition that age is not a disease, also the failure to recognize the richness of older women's lives; issues affecting women's work, retirement and pensions; the new multitasking grandparenting in response to myriad family and economic changes and the much neglected topic of friendships as keystones in women's lives.

Throughout I emphasized that much of women's aging is socially constructed; that is, it is largely culturally defined and enacted through the twin mechanisms of ageism and sexism. Women internalize these mechanisms which influence their images of themselves and instill unnecessary fears of aging. Far from having been eradicated, in the present era ageism appears to be increasing and taking new forms. Molly Andrews, discussing the growing pursuit of agelessness, reflects on the irony that people who practice ageism will one day join the group against which they are discriminating.[1] This is in contrast to those who are racist or sexist, meaning a racist Caucasian will not become Afro-American, nor will a male who practices sexism become a female. However, everybody gets older. Almost twenty-five years ago Eena Job, an Australian woman, deploring the effects of negative views of aging, described some women's response to ageist stereotypes, suggesting they were being anaesthetized into a more or less cheerful state of resignation.[2] Most mid-life women have moved a long way from cheerful resignation but still face important challenges. The big question is: what might we expect now that baby boom women are approaching their later lives? Will they capitalize on their strengths pushing for needed changes on their own behalf? And, if so, in what ways? How far will they go to remove the obstacles on their roadmaps, not only affecting themselves but also their daughters and granddaughters? Remember the cliché that men are more boisterous in their youth, becoming more conservative as they age, with women doing the reverse? I now examine several approaches to the question of whether or not baby boom women will engage in advocacy.

Will she or won't she?

Canadian analyst Charmaine Spencer, herself a boomer, asks: "Will Baby Boomers Become a Political Force as they Age?"[3] She notes first that baby boomers have been raised with high expectations regarding education, medicine and technology, citing the popular idea that they are not taking a back seat as they age, passively accepting the systems and roles of their parents and grandparents. Spencer argues, however, that their mere demographic numbers are not a sufficient ground upon which to base expectations of future activist involvement. She notes boomers' heterogeneity, their differing ages, economic and social positions. It is her feeling that, since the 1960s and 1970s, there has been little evidence of boomer activism. Looking at Canadian boomers, Spencer sees trends that suggest weakened social bonds, detachment and anomie rather than involvement. For example, with regard to such civic engagement as voting, she finds that voting is more important among older Canadians that among mid-life Canadians. A significant percentage of middle-aged boomers who did not vote suggests that they did not have confidence in the candidates. As Spencer puts it: "It is important to recognize that a malaise of discontent and a strong feeling that political participation is meaningless exists among many baby boomers."[4] This lack of confidence in politicians, is hardly surprising, having been much discussed in general. As one example of far too many, during the 1993 Federal election campaign, the candidate Jean Chretien promised to scrap or replace the Goods and Services Tax (GST). When he became Prime Minister, he did no such thing. In British Columbia, the Liberals promised new long-term beds for ailing seniors at election time, but once elected, began closing hospital beds. Looking at possible directions for boomer activism, Spencer points out that given increasing economic inequality, even if activism does occur it may not necessarily be progressive: "The more affluent (and also more influential) segment of the boomer generation may oppose redistributive politics."[5] She suggests that among the things needed for a more advocacy-directed boomer generation are an improved capacity to organize, balanced information for informed choices, and critical thinking. So the potential exists, but there needs to be a concerted effort to change public attitudes across the generations and to overcome the detachment presently felt. The US Presidential candidacy in 2008 between Barack Obama and Hillary Clinton certainly drew the attention of many who had previously not been involved, among them youth and ethnic minorities.

Along the same lines as Spencer, Robyn Stone, an American analyst asks: "Where Have all the Advocates Gone?" She looks back at her own efforts and notes that, twenty-five years later, just as the United States was about to experience the most significant demographic phenomenon in its history – the aging of the baby boomers – she finds that national advocacy for aging policies and programs seem to have lost their compass. Stone suggests several factors have contributed to a withering of advocacy for aging policies. Whereas in past decades, older people were viewed as deserving social support, now, with the projected numbers of aging boomers, older people are seen as either a market potential or budget busters draining public resources rather than as a wake-up call for advocacy. She finds that too many organizations are fighting for a slice of the pie, competing for scarce resources. As she wryly comments, "special interests have discovered aging," mostly in the health sectors.[6] Noting the persistence of ageism, finding it ironic that, just as we are about to experience the aging of the baby boom generation, ageism, in her opinion seems to be increased. She suggests a need to develop new strategies for aging advocacy-building coalitions, clarifying the message and training future aging advocates. She feels this is best done at the local level.

A similar perspective comes from the Australian Betsy Wearing, a health and fitness expert, who refers to the "dominant discourse" of ageism, which devalues older people and which is fostered through cultural representations (e.g. the media, language). She uses fitness as an interesting metaphor. While she notes the commodification of leisure in advanced industrial capitalism (the growth of a fitness industry) she sees it as an area of freedom that expresses itself through exercise and fitness. This offers an antidote to the ageist culture of degeneration and decline because it shows what midlife and older people can do, rather than what they can't.[7]

One final point is taken from Molly Andrews. Discussing "the new ageism" which, to her is the pursuit of agelessness, she cautions boomers not to fall into its trap, but rather focus on developmental possibilities which getting older affords. In her words: "If development is the project of a lifetime . . . then surely in a fundamental sense, age is an accomplishment, something one has worked long and hard at."[8] Rejection of the new ageism is an expression of personal resistance to an oppressive mould. Andrews speaks of the tension between change and continuity and suggests that we shift the centre of our thinking to the experiences of those who have been marginalized - older women. Though she doesn't discuss advocacy writ large, this idea of tension between change and continuity refers to a puzzling aspect of change, which I will address shortly.

Where does this leave us when it comes to attempting to fathom whether or not baby boom women will tackle difficulties they face? Which of the roads Spencer discusses in her sobering analysis will boomers take? Will they move further along the anomic path of detachment or will they move towards engagement? Will they follow Stone and attempt to act in small local groups to develop new strategies required by present realities? Will baby boom women shift the centre of attention from youth to later life? There are no easy answers. However, even recognizing that women are at a historical intersection, that women's increasing longevity is on a collision course with outworn concepts and policies-this is itself encouraging, and it is to be hoped, motivating. I now attempt to assess how things may play themselves out.

First, let's look at the view that baby boom women will not become advocates or activists. They may get lost in the pressures of the current climate of globalization and corporatization, the shrinking of the social welfare state, and the trend towards responsibility for self-sufficiently in later life now advancing towards individual responsibility rather than the state. This possibility certainly looms large. The respected American gerontologist Robert Binstock, writing about advocacy in this era of neo-conservatism, thinks that advocacy in the field of aging is a challenge, to say the least.

He notes the conservatism of national organizations that were formerly aging advocates (for example. the American Association of Retired Persons, which in his view has become quite moderate). He suggests that such advocacy grew out of the 1960s and 1970s and, in fact, has been out of style for a number of decades.[9]

The issues in the United States are different than those in Canada, especially given the possible changes to US social Security and the American privatized medical system, although one critic, as discussed in Chapter 4, has raised the red flag of possible pension changes in Canada.

Also as we have seen, most baby boom women are living in the fast-forward zone, with little time available doing both paid and unpaid work, (which one critic has called 'double unpaid overtime') while Spencer pointed out some are becoming more affluent and more removed from other women's realities. In other words, as we know, baby boomers are far from homogeneous.

A theme that ran through all the focus groups I organized involved the feeling that boomers belong to the "me" generation, that they want immediate gratification for themselves and their families, being self-involved and becoming more and more materialistic. A number of these older women felt that boomer's lives and the penchant among many towards consumerism is a far cry from the lives of previous generations. While boomers are generally portrayed in the media and elsewhere as having affected society by changing each stage of life as they live it, I noted in the Prologue that there are many contradictions in boomer lives, which suggests they are not all pulling in the same direction, and experiencing ages and stages of their lives differently from each other. Though their mass engagement in fitness and exercise and other preventative health practices will result in boomer women's healthier old age (certainly for the middle class). These perspectives indicate boomers' greater self-involvement and individual concerns which in turn suggests conservatism.

Yet it must be acknowledged that the fact that boomer women have more education, more workforce experience, more information, and better health than did many of the previous generations, all of which could certainly be the basis for more socially conscious engagement. They are clearly more assertive than the current older generation of women. The women who were involved in the women's movement of the 1960s and 1970s and who raised consciousness about rampant sexism and social injustice are the same women who are now in midlife and older. It's hard to imagine that they will sit back now and accept in their fifties and sixties what they would not accept in their twenties and thirties.

What might encourage women to become engaged? As mentioned above, Molly Andrews spoke about the tension between continuity and change. Such tensions become evident in the contradictions many women experience in their daily lives and may lead them to question how these conflicting experiences occur and are maintained.

Here are some possible situations: the contradiction between the lack of equity in the pay they receive and the work they do being connected to the large holes in the pension system which deprive many of a more secure old age; another, the contradiction between the lack of affordable daycare is connected to the now huge numbers of women in the workforce and dual-earner families; also the growing need to care for ailing parents and other elders is connected to the paucity of home care; the continuing interruption to work resulting from having unpaid family responsibilities connect to lost pension benefits; longevity and the possibility of later life chronic illness connects to the present inefficiencies of the public health system and the looming possibility of further privatization. In addition, professional women are still faced with a glass ceiling, which as a woman on a Canadian Broadcasting Corporation documentary pointed out, is not made of glass but rather of layers of men with power. However, Wallace Immen, writing in the *Globe and Mail*, January 26/08, finds that a number of women in highest paid, top executive positions in Canada had declined in the year 2007. Women university graduates still earn less than do male graduates.

These contradictions in boomer women's lives affect both those in the working class and those in the professional class, although the latter have more means.

Yet women frequently reinvent themselves, and all the ingredients seem to be present for effecting radical changes. Let's turn to the possibility of political engagement.

Setting the Table for the Twenty-First Century

Over and over we hear the phrases "on the table" and "off the table." These refer to which issues will be or will not be discussed within a variety of institutions, organizations, and policy makers. I now look at what needs to be 'on the table' for women in the twenty-first century.

Much is written on the involvement of women in Canadian politics, and there are several interesting considerations relevant to the activities of boomer women. Provincially in 1916, women got the vote in Manitoba, Saskatchewan, and Alberta; in 1917, they got it in Ontario, and British Columbia; 1918, in Nova Scotia; 1919, in New Brunswick; 1922, in Prince Edward Island; and in 1925, in Newfoundland. Quebec did not grant women the right to vote until 1940. In 1920, the Dominion Election Act gave women the same voting rights as men. Shamefully, Aboriginal women did not get the vote until 1960. For quite some time, women could not be appointed to the Senate because, before 1929, English Common Law declared that women were persons in matters of pains and penalties but not in matters of rights and privileges. It was not until October 18, 1929, that a group of women from Alberta known as the Famous Five – Nellie McClung, Henrietta Muir Edwards, Irene Parlby, Louise McKinney and Emily Murphy – forced Parliament to declare that women were indeed persons, and that they were eligible for appointment to the Senate.[10]

Instituted in 1909 by the Socialist Party of America, International Women's Day has been adopted by various countries throughout the world to mark the accomplishments of women and to foster women's rights. It was recognized by the United Nations in 1945 in the first international agreement to proclaim gender equality as a fundamental right. It is observed by many Canadian women who, with tongue in cheek, refer to it as Person's Day. Not being a "person" must have been quite a surprise to women working in factories, on farms, or in the home, raising families, making clothing and soap, growing, canning, and storing food. It is worth noting that Mother's Day, before today's greeting card pap, had radical origins as a powerful feminist call to end the war. Penned in the wake of the American Civil War in 1870, "A Mother's Day Proclamation" was written by Julia Ward Howe, and its opening line begins: "Arise, then, women of this day!"[11]

Following the federal election in June 2004, the Canadian House of Commons included sixty-five women, who occupied 21.1% of the three-hundred and eight seats. This percentage appears to be the norm. And, indeed, it is a far cry from 1957, for example, when the percentage of women elected in the two-hundred-sixty-five member Parliament was 0.8% (two women).[12] The Liberal government fell, and following the subsequent election of the Conservatives on January 23, 2006, sixty-four women or 20.7% were elected. In the 2008 election (Canada has had an election epidemic this decade) 68 women were elected to the House of Commons up from 64 in the previous election. Women will now occupy 22.1 percent of the 308 seats in the house compared to 21 percent in 2006. Yes, we have made gains. But taking fifty years to achieve well under one-quarter representation in Parliament is not exactly something to write home about. Equal Voice, a national advocacy group whose purpose is to get more women elected, hoped it might achieve at least one-third representation. It points out that Canada lags behind a number of European countries.[13] Equal Voice finds among the barriers facing women entering politics, are family responsibilities, having a less favourable financial position than men, and women being socialized to see politics as an unsuitable career. Non-partisan political advocacy groups in several provinces, called Women's Campaign Schools, hold sessions from time to time to train women who would like to run for political office. The treatment afforded Hillary Clinton's presidential candidacy, as discussed in Chapter one, was both sexist, ageist and replete with double standards. However the obverse side may be that US women have learned many political lessons among them that a strong, older woman was able to become a presidential candidate.

The subject of the number of women in governing bodies brings up a much discussed topic: will electing more women mean greater advocacy for women's issues? In other words, will elected women take pro-women positions? According to Jill Quadagno, "The real issue is whether female officeholders are likely to take different positions from males-positions that better represent women-and whether minorities bring a difference perspective to political debates."[14] Women who are elected are not of one voice. One thinks of Margaret Thatcher, the Iron Lady, who as prime minister of Great Britain ushered in an era of extreme conservatism, which certainly did not help older women or men. On the other hand, there was Golda Meier, the late Israeli prime minister. When she was informed that women were being assaulted by soldiers after dark and was advised to establish a curfew to get women off the streets, she responded by asking who was assaulting whom. She suggested that the curfew should apply to the soldiers, not to the women. Although these examples are not comparable, they certainly indicate very different perspectives. It should be made clear that numerous men both inside and outside Parliament regularly and strongly support needed change for women.

It is understood that whoever defines the debate will determine the policy agenda: what gets or doesn't get on the table. With regard to policies on aging, Spencer found that "Politically informed seniors have noted that it has become increasingly difficult, if not impossible to be present at the policy table. Often overjoyed to be heard at all, most seniors have not learned how to fight effectively against tokenism or how to effectively have issues reframed to better reflect seniors' circumstances."[15] If more women were to choose to become involved politically, then it is likely they would not accept tokenism–something that those women already elected strongly reject. Newly elected women would learn as have currently elected women, the strategies that define the debate, and the processes by which things get on the table. They would be familiar with how the media operates, and how to use such strategies as sound bytes and other methods of garnering headlines. The debate, of course will be seen differently by different elected women.

And Now for Something Completely Different, or the Full Monty

What kind of a world do most women really want? One in which:

- Earnings between men and women are equal

- Negative depictions of women in the media and elsewhere have been eradicated

- Language that demeans women is no longer used and such usage is considered to be hate-mongering, just as it is when it comes in the form of racist remarks

- The word senior is not in the vocabulary and,

with it, the belief that at age sixty-five we begin a downward slide

- The pension system recognizes and credits the value of caregiving and provides pensionable benefits for this work

- Homecare is affordable or subsidized and available for those who take or are given the responsibility of looking after frail elders

- Midlife and older women and men doing paid work get the same possibilities of further training and job promotions as do younger workers

Unfortunately there is no magic wand by which to wave this fantasy into being, but by way of starting, I suggest the following: a new three Rs.

Three Rs: Resenting, Resisting, and Reconstructing

Resenting

There is no shortage of items for this category but it is possible to direct resentment into positive channels. Tackling ageism is certainly one of these. Take, as one instance, greeting cards that feature hateful caricatures of older women. When you see one, simply ask yourself: "Would a similar greeting card be acceptable if it depicted a visible minority in this fashion?" If the answer is no, then don't buy it, and tell the store manager why you are doing so.

Women are not encouraged to display anger or resentment; rather, some are "anaesthetized into cheerful acceptance." Not always cheerful to be sure. Consider the following case history.

Case History

Anne followed all the rules by which she and other older women were socialized. She worked before she got married, then stayed at home to raise her children. In every possible way she was a model wife (at least from society's perspective). The house was immaculate, clothing duly washed and ironed, tasty meals prepared and served to a waiting (but not helpful) family. Everybody's needs were met and supported, and she rarely raised her voice. She also suffered from headaches. Her husband was a fairly prominent man in the community, and Anne found time to do volunteer work in organizations which were working for worthwhile causes. In his late sixties, Anne's husband began to ail, was in poor health for a number of years, and died in his late seventies. Shortly thereafter people began to notice a change in her behavior. She seemed to establish her own agenda, was less soft-spoken and uncharacteristically expressed opinions openly. In her late seventies she needed a hip replacement, following which she went to therapy at a hospital fairly close to her home, but to which she could not drive because of her recovering hip. If she couldn't get a ride she took taxis. One late and dreary winter afternoon, having finished at the hospital, she called for a taxi which failed to show up. She called several times but no taxi. Tired, uncomfortable and exasperated, she called a local paper. She told them she was a senior and explained her circumstances in no uncertain terms. A reporter arrived with a photographer and the next day Anne's picture was on the front page, where she denounced the lack of transportation for persons with her needs.

Did this change the world? Certainly not, but it was a changed Anne, who learned, late in life that swallowing anger was no longer acceptable. It is a fair wager that her headaches disappeared. If there is a moral in this story for boomer and younger women, it is to transform resentment into action by giving it a voice.

Ever heard of dancing dogs? Many years ago the American writer Cynthia Ozick wrote about what she termed dancing dogs, meaning that a performing dog is admired not because it is dancing well but, rather because it is dancing at all. This metaphor, borrowed like so much else from Samuel Johnson, can be duly applied to the accomplishments of older people. How many times have there been headlines such as: "Man, 77, Climbs Alpine Peak" or "Ninety-one year-old woman, Retired Academic, Still tutors Graduate Students" or "Grandmother, 80, Goes Whitewater Rafting." Why should these depictions be resented? Because what the media are doing is showing that these people are remarkable "for their age." They are expressing the view that these people are exceptional, portraying them as lovable freaks. The point is that those so portrayed are NOT remarkable for their age: they are normal for their age. Active, energetic midlife and older people are the norm, not the exception. To portray them otherwise is to be ageist. Whether the story or headline editors and TV producers recognize it or not, they are presenting a view based on the belief that older people are somehow diminished, or, if not, then they should be. Dissenting e-mails, phone calls, letters to editors might encourage some rethinking, suggesting to them that, in an era of population aging, this is not the way to go. One can think of those in their eighties and nineties who are making or made outstanding contributions: Kenneth Galbraith, Pablo Picasso, Arturo Toscannini, Jane Jacobs, Pablo Casals, Georgia O'Keefe, Jimmy Carter, Nelson Mandela, Simon Wiesenthal Therese Casgraine, and the Cuban musical group *Buena Vista Social Club*.

Resisting

Two evocative book titles were mentioned earlier: *Learning to be Old* and *Declining to Decline*. Both point to how debilitating and self-destructive it is for midlife women and older women to internalize the cultural imperatives of a society that is youth-obsessed and dismissive of older women. Gullette expresses this vividly when she refers to a book title to which she took exception: *How Did I Get to be Forty and Other Atrocities*. "I got to be forty by not dying beforehand, and damn if I'm going to consider this an atrocity. The real atrocity is cultural and economic depreciation of women (or men) who are 'past' youth."[16] We've seen how troubling it is for some women to resist the youth culture in which they are embedded.

Does this mean that effective resistance is impossible? Absolutely not. Resistance is the opposite of acquiescence, and women have demonstrated this dissatisfaction in numerous constructive ways. However, many find resistance difficult, especially to begin with. So here are some lighter approaches that may ease entering the resistance mode:

- Take a few counter-cultural steps, try not doing what you are expected to do. Instead, make a list of Resistance Resolutions (think of them as spirited New Year's Resolutions). You might

include on this list such things as "saying no."
For example, when you are asked to mind a child
at the time your favourite TV show comes on,
just say no. And don't feel guilty. If someone is
trying to make you feel guilty, that tells you more
about them than it does about yourself. Think of
some other things to which you might say no.

• Try to stop saying "I'm sorry." Women often
apologize for a range of things that are not their
responsibility. In my own case, the "I'm sorry"
epiphany came some years ago. I was at an
airport, rushing past a row of seated people,
when I tripped. Thinking I had stumbled over
someone's foot I said "I'm sorry" without even
thinking. Then I looked and saw that I had
tripped over a large umbrella that someone had
placed on a seat and was sticking way out into
the aisle. It's fine to say I'm sorry if you have
done something you are sorry about, but not
otherwise. Make a list of things you can say in
situations where you're accustomed to saying
you're sorry unnecessarily. For example, instead
of saying "I'm sorry dinner is late" try "dinner will
take a few minutes" or say why it is late.

• Avoid such phrases as "I'm having a senior's
moment." This undergirds the cultural view of

older people as being somewhat senile. We all get distracted at times and this can manifest itself as confusion. We all also have occasional memory loss. How many times do young people lock themselves out of the car or house? Do we refer to them as having "an adolescent's moment"? Think of how many times younger family members or friends lost keys or glasses? Of course some older people are more susceptible than others, but such loss occurs differently to different people. It may not occur at all. The brain responds to being challenged by new learning and mental exercises like solving difficult crossword puzzles. Now there are video games designed to assist with memory retention. One person noted that memory is not "lost," we simply need to learn to gain access to it in different ways. Think of how much information is jammed into our heads daily, especially in this technological age. Forgetting something or experiencing moments of distraction does not mean we are fast-tracking down the road to dementia. What other phrases do you think you might stop using?

• This next one is harder. Many midlife and older women don't want their age to be known, and within our current ageist context this is easily understood. One woman admits to turning her driver's licence face down because it is the only one of a number of identifying cards which states our age. Many feel that calendar years are not the valid measure of anyone's talents or capabilities. One of my focus group women in her late sixties stated: "I'm far more competent now that when I was thirty." Do you think you should hide your age? If so, why, and if not, why?

- Let's consider "humor". Someone asks an older person what her name is. She hesitates and then says irritably: "Do you have to know right now?" Such jokes are fine among peers. Ethnic and other minority groups certainly make jokes about themselves; this does no harm, in fact it functions to express group solidarity. But with ageist humor as widespread as it is, then one must ask: "Am I making fun of older people and/or demeaning them in any way?" It is hard to resist telling funny stories. What is your approach to this type of humor?

- Last in the resistance "to do's" is joining groups that are working to make change. There are numerous groups which women join, both formal and informal, that are working towards bringing about change in Canada and elsewhere.

Some of the issues that are currently high on the agenda are the environment, climate change, violence against women and elders, war, poverty, hunger (food banks, for example) housing and homelessness, mental health and social justice in general. Many women participate in political organizations, unions, academic, and community organizations. Through this activism, the needs of women are frequently reported and made visible. It is a long time since newspapers have had "women's sections" devoted to recipes and household hints. It has been made clear to newspapers that women are not a separate species having no interest in the world outside of families and kitchens.

However, not many of these multidimensional groups focus upon the situations of older women. Their issues rarely make it to "the table" or to public consciousness. There are some community-based exceptions one of which is Canadian and quite remarkable, a group known as the Raging Grannies. Its members have published a book with the wonderful title *Off Our Rockers*. In the words of Allison Acker and Betty Brightwell, who started it eighteen years ago in Victoria, British Columbia: "Once we were invisible. Like all older women we were expected to fade into the background along with our looks, our health, our income, and our importance to society. But not any more . . . a group of women . . . who decided to break the stereotype of nice but negligible grandmothers by becoming outrageous . . . we were out to shock . . . would dress up as crazy old ladies in extravagant hats to get the attention . . . and then we would rattle the cages of those who, we felt, were destroying our world . . . we would go where we were not invited and sing out loud what was not supposed to be said. We would be guerilla singers and we would change the world."[17] They recognize they haven't changed the world, however, "we've ruffled a few feathers, gotten a lot of media attention, annoyed many citizens and delighted others." There are few Canadians who haven't heard of them, seen them in their ridiculous hats, shawls, singing familiar songs to which they've written lyrics relating to the specific event they are sending up. The raging granny concept has spread to more than sixty groups, stretching across Canada and the United States and reaching into the United Kingdom, Europe, and even Australia. There are some similarly oriented American groups one comprised of six friends who spray paint "Avenge Ageism," on whatever seems appropriate; or a group called Guerilla Matrons, which defaces billboards advertising products using the images of anorexic teen age girls.

It is interesting to note that the Grannies' ranks are mostly middle-class, educated, most of whom do not otherwise engage in bizarre behavior (at least not in public). Hopefully taking off from stereotypical hatted, shawled and gloved grannies will soon be out of date, if it isn't already, given current midlife women "grandboomers." A small exploratory study by Adler et al. found that older adults are increasingly addressing issues facing their communities and larger society. Respondents who were social activists had higher educational levels and a concern for 'generativity', that is, support for upcoming generations.[18]

There are many less flamboyant groups than the Grannies or Guerilla Matrons, some of which are community based like Vancouver's Women Elders in Action (WE'ACT), which has published a booklet about Canadian women and the pension system. The United States has the Older Women's League (OWL) and the already mentioned American Association of Retired Person (AARP), Canada has the Status of Women and the Canadian Association for the Fifty Plus and Seniors (formerly CARP); the latter has a section devoted to advocacy. Also the National Council of Women along with the Older Women's Network, devoted to addressing barriers facing mid-life and older women, including economic security, and no doubt numerous others. Most now have internet portals. British women have the "Hen Co-op" which is dedicated to growing old 'disgracefully', meaning they should seek to please themselves rather than abide by traditional passivity of the "shoulds" and "oughts." The British analyst and feminist Sara Arber comments on how baby boom women, being better educated and more equality oriented, may achieve the Hen Co-op's goals.[19] Being active on their own behalfs, she notes, will mean balancing choices and constraints, the latter including adequate resources, their caring responsibilities and their own health and functional abilities.

Reconstruction

A very tall order indeed, and likely the one that is most challenging as it means confronting power structures head on. A basic question is, how do we shift the agenda and get the concerns of midlife and older women moved from the margins to the centre, from invisibility to recognition? I've noted a number of formal and informal groups, some of which are devoted to women's concerns and many of which are found in the political and activist arena. This is all to the good. However it seems that too few of such groups are shining the spotlight on midlife and older women or the issues raised in this book, while women are increasing in number and forming the bulk in population aging. Efforts made on their behalf such as their future financial security will be not only be important to them but to women of all ages. Some of the challenges are enormous. For example, should energy be directed towards a small change to the Canada/Quebec Pension Plan to allow a three-year dropout period to those providing eldercare, as suggested in Chapter 4, let alone pensionable credits for that work which continues to grow? Once we put our minds to it, any number of possibilities for manageable change will come into view. Issues are not in short supply.

"Here's Looking at You, Kid"

This is what Humphrey Bogart said to Ingrid Bergman in *Casablanca*. Given the enormous roles that the media, especially TV, play in influencing and shaping attitudes towards women as they age, it is more than time to stare back, much as media watch groups do, but to do so now through the eyes of midlife women. One study of the media and aging conducted by the Harvard School of Public Health-Metlife Foundation points out "how entertainment and news media work in association with public policy and marketing concerns to reflect and influence the category 'old age' as boomers strain at its boundary."[20] At the same time as younger and still younger people are pervasive marketing targets, the aging population is increasingly being recognized in the "grey as gold" markets. Corporate advertisers are reaching out to boomers and their potential spending power. There are articles on the internet with titles such as "More marketers target boomers' eyes, wallets." Or "Millions of wrinkles, billions of dollars." Some of the products being pushed are new drugs, financial, and investment possibilities, gated-community residences with golf courses aimed at pre-retirees and those already retired. Given the power of corporate television, not only are attitudes about older people influenced, but possibly policies. After all, policy wonks also watch TV and read newspapers and magazines, and the advertising they see suggests that most older people are well off with secure futures. This is not the case.

The pervasiveness of television during the past fifty years, and its hold on millions, possibly billions of viewers around the world, is a historic technological first. There are now several generations who have grown up with television, as well as with films, videos and games. It is unlikely – in fact probably impossible, given the market-driven capitalist, globalized world in which we live – that the power of the corporate media will loosen its hold on our minds. This not to say that women shouldn't do whatever can be done to lessen its damaging effects. It may be a David and Goliath scenario, but "little permed women" (a phrase used by an ageist male columnist) have shown their strength before. The time is ripe, indeed overripe to move towards reconstructing these unacceptable representations. Those in the women's movement in the 1970s started media watch groups to critique the sexism prevalent at that time. They were effective in bringing attention to this issue in its many forms. Small groups of mid-life women resentful of the misrepresentations can find innovative approaches to deal with ageism. Midlife media watchdog groups devoted to lessening ageism might turn the tide, just as did those devoted to lessening sexism in the recent past.

And midlife women will be the majority. Size and gender count.

In the three years since I started writing this book, in fact in 2005, encouraging evidence has made itself felt that some change is blowing in the wind. For example, as noted, protests against the prevalence of wafer-thin models, which seriously damage teen - aged women's self-image and their health, are making themselves felt in Israel, Spain, and some other countries. And Helen Mirren, the British actor, won the Oscar at the age of sixty at the 2007 Academy Awards. And, according to James Adams, writing in the *Globe and Mail CTV* on February 12, 2008, *More*, a magazine aimed at women forty years or older, has become an instant Canadian success story, with circulation of almost 125 000 since its launch the previous year. A most promising development has been made by the Canadian media mogul, as he is called, Moses Znaimer , who in February of 2008, coined the word "Zoomers" to describe the over fifty age demographic. This will be the name of a magazine, plus a multi media strategy, including internet advocacy on behalf of the current aging generation.

As the new executive director of C.A.R.P. (see above), he urges societal change in its attitude to age and aging, in a culture which overemphasizes youth. Yet another whiff of change comes from a US group "Women's Voices for Change" has named a popular syndicated columnist Liz Smith, the "Anne Richards Trouble Maker in Residence," named after the much-admired activist, the late Anne Richards, former Governor of Texas. In one of her columns, Smith asked whether America is ready to be led by "retiring boomers, a majority of whom are menopausal and post-menopausal." [21] All to the good.

In addition, to these new encouraging signs of change, and perhaps the most substantive to date because it targets older women, has come from the two studies by Dove beauty campaigns, discussed in Chapter 2. The first, *The Real Truth About Beauty*, released in February, 2004 found that only 1% of Canadian women and only 2% of women worldwide consider themselves beautiful: a frightening testimony to the power of youth-drenched corporate advertising. Dove's second study, *Beauty Comes of Age* released February, 2007, found that 86% of the women questioned, aged fifty to sixty-four, were happy with their age and their bodies, but over 90% felt that media and society's portrayals misrepresented them.

A number of them allowed themselves to be photographed in the nude for the 2007 study, declaring they were proud of their bodies. This study evoked a surprisingly large reaction, including a 10 page insert in the *Globe and Mail* on March 8th, 2007 (International Women's Day!) devoted entirely to the 2007 Dove campaign. It featured articles by a number of prominent women who wrote variously about a "new era of maturity" with topics about mid-life women on health, sexuality, resilience and independence. The insert, including the photographed women, also featured comments made by everyday women in response to the study, mostly favourable.

This huge response raises a number of issues and some interesting questions. It made clear that the mid-life women they questioned were fine with their age, pleased with their bodies and resentful of being misinterpreted in popular imagery. Although Dove's campaign was market targeted to introduce a new line of products for baby-boom women, featuring a Pro-Aging slogan, it has triggered a remarkable response. Somehow, it became a catalyst encouraging discussion of other positive aspects of boomer women's lives, rarely heard. In fact, it seems to have done in a very short time what numbers of women writers and analysts have written and talked about for years (witness the number of them referred to in this book alone).

Is this a contradiction? Is it a beneficial unintended consequence? The studies were thoughtfully designed and conducted. They accomplished a great deal in the portrayals of midlife women, revealing their thoughts and attitudes including their resentment of misrepresentative images. Perhaps other advertisers (there is already one beauty product copycat at the time of this writing) and the media will examine their own attitudes and advertising content. The Dove campaign could motivate mid-life and older women to engage in ways to further these findings. In the fifties, there were Tupperware parties which spread like wildfire. Women in the 21st Century, given technological advances, might innovate strategies far beyond living-room get-togethers (although these are not to be mocked) to talk about moving forward with the studies' findings.

A number of organizations already exist on the net, for example the *National Association of Baby Boom Women*, an American effort which dedicates itself to "Empowering Women to Explore and Live Their Passions."[22]

A 2005 American book by Jennifer Baumgardner and Amy Richards entitled *Grassroots: A Field Guide for Feminist Activism* sounds promising. While it offers sound information and advice regarding activist women, consideration of activism in relation to older women, boomers or otherwise, to aging or to seniors did not make it on their radar screen.

One final point with respect to reconstruction and advocacy among boomer women. As previously stated, there is a belief that women become more activist as they age. This leads to the question as to what circumstances would prompt women to become active? Again, not an easy question. Several of the Raging Grannies to whom I posed this question, reflected that almost all of their members had been activists throughout their lives, supporting change in a number of major area (e.g. the environment). Few became activists for the first time in later life. I addressed a more specific question when I interviewed a prominent, older Canadian women, Margaret Fulton, a life long feminist, one of the first women to become president of a Canadian university (The University of Mount St. Vincent in Nova Scotia) and the recipient of numerous awards and distinctions. I asked if women, as they age and become aware of situations that require restructuring, would this motivate them to do something about them? Her reply was, "Yes, absolutely." She went on to say that things happen in life no matter at what age, and that some of those things will bring an epiphany. For example, if a women is deserted by a husband or partner, then she has to face many things, such as finances, child support, visiting and custody. Or, if an older person becomes frail and her caregiver daughter tries to arrange for a homemaker, then she is exposed to a set of structures that were previously unfamiliar to her personally. In Fulton's view, such experiences familiarize women with the numerous contradictions and discriminations they face, and she believes that this could motivate activism. In other words, once a woman encounters a structural barrier that prohibits her from getting the help she needs, she may want to do something about it. When bad things happen to us it is only human to then want to strike back.

Back to the Future (or the Beginning, or . . .)

Canada is a rich and wonderful country, with strong democratic values and respect for human rights. It has many institutions which Canadians hold in high regard, among them its public health care and pension systems. These among other values play a huge role in people's lives, and given the large numbers of boomer cohorts, will certainly continue to do so in the future. One of the things which motivated me to write this book is the knowledge that over 37% of older unattached Canadian women live at or below the current poverty line. This fact reflects only one among numerous issues concerning women as they age which are discussed in academic journals, books, articles and talks. I believe these analyses and ideas warrant being made available to a greater number of women. As I have already discussed, midlife boomer women are about to occupy or are already occupying new stages of their lifecourse. In selecting the topics for this book, my purpose was to examine various familiar situations in order to trumpet women's many strengths. As well to think about how certain issues affected their lives, some of them barriers precluding the achievement of social and financial security in later life. The idea that aging is more culturally than biologically determined struck me as a particularly critical concept. As Margaret Gullette reminds us, revulsion towards aging is not innate, it is learned. I wanted to encourage yet-to-be older women to reject the negative stereotypes to which they are exposed and to minimize their fears of aging. I wanted to encourage mid-life boomer women to celebrate their many strengths and accomplishments, now and to come. I wanted to suggest that, despite inevitable difficulties, older age can be one of the most fulfilling times of women's lives.

I have attempted to show how women's aging is socially constructed, how this has damaged many women of my generation, and how this might continue to play itself out among the growing numbers of boomer women. My concern was to try and determine whether the present widespread negative social, cultural and economic practices affecting women were simply going to continue. How might they be amenable to change? Was the poverty and late-life insecurity that now blemishes many older women's lives going to keep on happening in perpetuity? What, in the face of global restructuring and downsizing, are the chances of creating opposition? How do we challenge the intertwining of the corporate media with the corporate health while social safety nets are being cut to accommodate the pervasive gods of bottom lines? These are major dilemmas.

I support getting rid of the word "senior" because it suggests an age-segregated model of aging. It presents "seniors" as a group that is separate from others and no longer capable of further development. It clearly misrepresents the new realities of aging, since the great majority of those over sixty are energetic, contributing citizens. What's wrong with "older persons" or "mature persons"? The Harvard study I noted above found the current language of aging to be obsolete, to be an impediment to change because it oversimplifies many complexities. Of course, so does the term "boomers": probably even more so, given the huge numbers, diversity and contradictions within this category. *Mea culpa.* I didn't know how else to approach it, given the word's popularity and omnipresence.

I struggled with the nature of change itself. Change happens. What are its properties in relation to coming generations of older women and how does change at the individual level shift in order to become change at the collective level? Think of smoking. By "naming it" as a health problem and by creating educational programs (including many that are shown on TV) the incidence of smoking has been cut dramatically in many countries, despite constant advertising on the part of giant corporate cigarette industries – yet another contradiction. What started as individual change became a collective change. Is a similar process possible with regard to addressing the present neglect of older and soon-to-be-older women? I believe that it is.

I must offer another *mea culpa* for the many topics I have not been able to address: enormously important topics such as housing, transportation, immigrant women, and Aboriginal women. I have been criticized for having a case of "Atlasitis," that is, carrying the whole world on my shoulders. Being older (and wiser?) now, I decided that in this book I would only carry a part of the world on my shoulders. On the occasion of my eightieth birthday, my kids gave me a T-shirt inscribed as follows: "If you can remain calm, you don't have all the facts." They were tweaking my constant concerns about large issues. Certainly this attitude formed part of the motivation to write this book. There is a common belief that women who live to be eighty have learned to be flexible and to change with the times. I agree with this. But I would add that women not only change with the times, but have a history of changing the times. When Betty Friedan wrote *The Feminine Mystique* in 1963 she addressed what she called "the problem that has no name": something she saw affecting many women in suburbia, women who were living outwardly model, normal lives but who were inwardly dissatisfied and depressed, constantly swallowing the tranquilizers that the doctors of the time so freely prescribed. The response to her book was nothing short of astounding. Friedan had pushed dormant buttons, the response was world shaking. More recently, in 2006, the outstanding American feminist and social analyst, Carroll Estes, remarks on the abundance of many academic voices calling for profound social change.[23] "Yet" she notes "the reality is that there is little old-age policy and nascent, if any grassroots feminist social movement activity building on the critiques." She calls this "the missing feminist revolution" in social policy and aging.

The women's movement of the 1960's and 1970's was fractious and diverse. It, too named many issues that were no longer to be tolerated, such as rampant sexism. Opposition to racism also came to the fore during these times and "Black is beautiful" became a rallying cry for African-Americans. Gay Liberation was born with the Stonewall riots in 1969 and came of age in the 1970s. Naming all these issues gave each of them a voice.

The women's movement literally changed women's worlds. Women's studies courses were established at universities and colleges, no easy task in the face of heated opposition. The outpouring of research, books and other writing that have come out of women's studies has literally rewritten the history of women. My generation of older women had never seen a female news anchor or even heard a female voice reading the news on the radio. Nor did we see women delivering the mail, being police officers, soldiers, electricians, plumbers, dentists, doctors, or lawyers. Sometimes these remarkable changes are taken for granted by those who are currently young, many of whom are unaware of the extent and cost of the resistance that brought them about.

It is well to remember some of the successful strategies that the women's movement employed, foremost among them being the banner call of "the personal is political." This urged women to look at their own personal situations, the things they felt were holding them back, their unexpressed resentment, and then to connect these events to larger social structures. Under the rubric of "consciousness raising," women started meeting in small groups in each others homes and elsewhere, started talking to each other and soon realized that most of them shared the same dissatisfactions. They followed up such disclosures in a variety of ways, organizing, holding meetings, writing and speaking out about them. All kinds of unpleasant discoveries were made and acknowledged for what they were. For example, female university students who joined with male students in campus groups, the idea being to change education's top-down authoritarian administration, found that "the men made the decisions, while the women made the coffee." They clearly recognized that the men were not sharing power with women equitably, even in small groups, let alone power structures. Women had to take power themselves. And they did. They found their voices. And now we need to recognize that, in the words of Margaret Gullette, "Age (specifically age as decline) can no longer be omitted from the lists of the great categorical oppressions."[24] There is some current envisioning of initiating studies of ageism-not studies of aging, or about aging, but adding ageism as a category and seeing it as important as sexism and racism.

Has the time for conscious-raising and activism on behalf of older women finally arrived? I think it most definitely has. But it is for boomer women to decide what to do about this.

Consciousness-raising would have a different name now, and it could take new forms, forms amenable to new technologies. Boomer women working in groups, in the community, in politics and in unions and on the net could urge putting older women's concerns "on the table." Small groups might grow into larger entities: witness the Raging Grannies.

The internet offers undreamed of potential for the proliferation of ideas and the joining of virtual hands. Those confronting the barriers that many growing older women are facing, and will continue to face, will have numbers on their side: over the next couple of decades four million-plus Canadian boomer women will join the ranks of those over sixty-five.

But numbers alone don't translate into street power. There is, as yet, no older women's movement. It has to be named, given a voice and made visible. If this were to happen, then it would be folly for politicians to ignore it.

We must remember what the gay and lesbian (LGBT) communities have taught us. They made their needs a street issue, and made sure that the injustices they faced (and, indeed, continue to face) became the stuff of everyday consciousness. One result of this is that same-sex marriage is now legal in Canada. Gay Pride days and parades are now common throughout North America and Europe, are applauded by thousands, indeed hundreds of thousands of straight people who line the streets, cheer, and clap. One of the most resilient LGBT slogans is: "We're here, we're queer, get used to it."

Perhaps older women could try: "We're older, we're bolder, deal with it." Why not?

As the feminist writer Gloria Steinem said twenty-five years ago "Someday an army of old gray women will take over the earth."[25] Now seems as good a time as any for mid-life women to bring this about. In fact, now is an exceptionally good time.

References

1. Molly Andrews, "The Seductiveness of Agelessness," *Aging and Society* 19 (1999): 303.

2. Eena Job, *Eighty Plus: Outgrowing the Myths of Old Age* (Queensland: University of Queensland Press, 1984).

3. Charmaine Spencer, "Grey Power in Canada: Will Baby Boomers Become a Political Force as They Age?" *Gerontology Research Centre News*, Simon Fraser University, 11 (2003): 1-5.

4. Ibid., 3.

5. Ibid., 4.

6. Robyn Stone, "Where Have All the Advocates Gone?" *Generations* 28, 1 (Spring 2004): 61.

7. Betsy Wearing, "Leisure and Resistance in an Aging Society," *Leisure Studies* 14 (1995): 263-79.

8. Andrews, "The Seductiveness of Agelessness," 310.

9. Robert H. Binstock, "Advocacy in an Era of New Conservatism: Responses of National Aging Organizations," Generations 28, 1 (Spring 2004): 49-54.

10. "What Is Person's Day?," <http://womenet.ca/news/php?show&1907> (accessed June 30, 2005).

11. <http://www.uoakron.edu.geography/people/klosterman> (accessed May 13, 2004).

12. Elections Canada, "Federal Election Update: How Many Women in Parliament? 2004-06-30," <http://www.womenet.ca/news/php?show&1907> (accessed April 2, 2005). See also <http://www.equalvoice.ca/womenelected.pdf> for January 23, 2006 election (accessed February 23, 2006). "Equal Voice: Federal Election Results 2008." <http://www.straightgoods.ca/Election2008/ViewNews.cfm?Ref=77> (Accessed November 18, 2008).

13. Ibid.

14. Jill Quadagno, *Aging and the Lifecourse: An Introduction to Social Gerontology*, 2nd Ed. (Boston: McGraw Hill, 2002), 455.

15. Charmaine Spencer, "Grey Power in Canada: Part One," *Gerontology Research Centre News*, Simon Fraser University, August 19, 2000, 5-8.

16. Margaret Morganroth Gullette, *Declining to Decline: Cultural Combat and the Politics of the Midlife* (Charlottesville and London: University Press of Virginia, 1997), 92.

17. Allison Acker and Betty Brightwell, eds. *Off Our Rockers and into Trouble* (Victoria: Touch Wood Editions, 2004), xi-xii passim.

18. Geri Adler, Jennifer Schwartz and Michael Kuskowsky, "An Exploratory Study of Older Adults' Participation in Civic Action," Clinical Gerontologist 31, 2. 2007, 65-75

19. Sara Arber, "Gender and Later Life: Change, Choice and Constraints" in John A. Vincent, Chris R. Phillipson and Murna Downs. Eds. *The Futures of Old Age* London: Sage Publications, 2006. 54.

20. "Shifting Images of Aging in the Media," in *Reinventing Aging: Baby Boomers and Civic Education*, Harvard School of Public Health-Metlife Foundation, Initiative on Retirement and Civic Engagement, Centre for Health Communications, Harvard School of Public Health, 2004.

21. <http://www.womensvoicefor change.org/>

22. National Association of Baby Boom Women, *NABBW News*, April 2007 <http://www.nabbw.com> (accessed April 7, 2007).

23. Carroll Estes, "Critical feminist Perspectives, Aging and Social Policy" in Jan Baars et al., Eds. *Aging, Globalization and Inequality: The New Critical Gerontology*, Society and Aging Series, John Hendricks, Series Editor (Amityville, N.Y.: Baywood Publishing Company, Inc., 2006).

24. Margret Morganaroth Gullette, *Aged by Culture* (Chicago and London: University of Chicago Press, 2004), 122.

25. Gloria Steinem, *Outrageous Acts and Everyday Rebellions*, 2nd Ed. (New York: Henry Holt and Company, 1995), 236 (first published in 1983).

Endnote

aglady or Powerhouse? was written shortly before the huge global and financial meltdown, though there are some references to it. The consequences of these events will not be known until some future time. However, among other topics, the book argues the financial vulnerability of many midlife and older women's lives. It is likely that their late life security may now be even less secure. This makes it more important that midlife women concern themselves with some of the empowering measures the book discusses, on their own behalfs and for those who follow them.

Appendices

Appendix 1:
Compassionate Care

Canada has recently acquired Compassionate Care Benefits of up to six weeks to attend to a gravely ill family member. For more information refer to Employment Insurance (EI) Compassionate Care Benefits. There are some enlightened employers who recognize their employees' need for time off to attend to such family responsibilities. This also occurs more typically in collective agreements with public employers, who have "special leave" provisions.

Appendix 2:
The Canada Pension System

Canada's pension system consists of a mix of public and private components. It has three major parts, and thus is commonly referred to as being three-tiered.

The first tier

The first tier involves the Old Age Security (OAS), the Guaranteed Income Supplement (GIS) and the

Allowance (ALW), (formerly referred to as the spouse's allowance). The OAS is a flat-rate amount of money available to almost all persons in Canada over the age of sixty-five, with certain residency requirements. Funding comes from the general tax base, and until 1989 the OAS could be considered to be universal; however, since then it has been 'clawed back' so that wealthier recipients, those who's income is over $64 718 in 2008 have to repay 15% of the difference between that amount and their income .It should be noted that the clawback is not indexed. As of January-March 2008 the OAS average monthly benefit was $476.36. This amount is indexed against inflation, based on the consumer price index (CPI). The benefits are income taxable. Around 95% of Canadians aged sixty-five and over receive the OAS.

The GIS is payable to OAS recipients who have a low income or no other source of income. It is income-tested and is not taxable. It is paid monthly to single persons, or to the spouse of common-law partner of a non-pensioner, or an allowance recipient. As of January-March 2008 the average monthly benefit was from $437.37 to $634.02 according to which category is applicable. GIS benefits are reduced by fifty cents for every dollar of non-OAS income. Please note that same-sex common law partners have the same benefits and obligations as do opposite-sex common-law partners.

The Allowance and Allowance for survivors (ALW) is also subject to an income test, is paid monthly to a spouse or common-law partner or to a survivor. It is designed to help surviving persons and couples living on the pension of only one spouse or common-law partner, if they are between the ages of sixty and sixty-four. One must apply for each of the first tier benefits.

The second tier

The second tier of the Canadian pension system is the retirement pension, which is referred to as the Canada and Quebec Pension Plans (C/QPP), referred to hereafter as the (CPP) which was instituted in 1966. Contributions are compulsory for all paid workers over the age of eighteen, including those who are self-employed. The CPP is a pay-as-you-go plan, meaning that its funds accrue from its mandatory contributions. It is calculated on the basis of defined benefits. Contributions are made by both the employer and the employee, but those who are self-employed must pay the full amount (i.e. of both the employer and the employee). These contributions are taxable deductions. Annual benefits are indexed against inflation. Quebec administers its own plan – the QPP – which in all major respects is coordinated with the CPP. Certain reforms were put in place in 1997 by an Act of Parliament to make the C/QPP sustainable in the face of population aging which included raising contributions to 9.9%: half from employers and half from employees. There was also a CPP Investment Board, independent of the CPP established in 1998, which is charged with 'prudent and responsible' investment of CPP's fund. At December 31, 2006 the fund stood at $110.8 billion. The earnings of these investments are also part of the funding base.

In addition to retirement benefits, the CPP also provides survivor's benefits, orphan's or child's benefits, and disability benefits. There is also a seven-year drop out provision (Child Rearing Provision), meaning a parent who stays home to raise a child up to the age of seven does not have the lack of contributions during this period counted for final benefits. The contribution rates based on 25% of the average industrial wage (which in 2008 is approximately $44 900). The OAS was designed to provide about 15% of retirement income, and together with the CPP, to replace forty per-cent of pre-retirement income. There is a ceiling for maximum benefits at age sixty, which as of January 1, 2008 was $884.58. It is important to note that the CPP does not get its funds from the general tax base; rather, its administration and payouts come from the contribution base (i.e. the contributions made from both employers and employees) which are taxable. This fact is not emphasized sufficiently, and this often leaves the impression that benefits come from the general tax base as they do for the OAS and the rest of the first tier of the pension system.

The CPP's individual retirement benefits are based on a formula that, in turn, is based on earnings and time spent in the labor force. Pension benefits are available for persons who retire early, from age sixty to sixty-four, reducing the amount received by .05% per month, which could mean a reduction of 30% of benefits for persons retiring at age sixty. Similarly, people can pay benefits up to age seventy, which would afford them a further increase of .05% per month, or 30% of their benefits if they work until they are seventy. Once one starts getting the CPP pension, no further contributions can be made. The CPP also allows for pension credits to be split between spouses/common partners either upon divorce or retirement.

The Third Tier

The third tier of the Canadian pension system consists of the registered retirement savings plan (RRSP), the registered pension plan (RPP), a group RRSP and a registered retirement investment fund (RRIF) which was raised to age seventy-one in the 2007-08 budget.

The RRSP is a registered retirement savings plan, meaning it is registered with the Canada Customs and

Revenue Agency for tax purposes, as well as with the federal and provincial pension regulatory authority, as are all of the third-tier plans. The RRSP is a voluntary individual savings plan, allowing individuals to contribute to their retirement savings. There is a limit based on 18% of the previous tax year to a fixed maximum in 2008 of $20 000 rising to $22 000 in 2010. RRSP's are a tax shelter (deferred taxation), meaning that individuals who put money into them do not have to pay taxes until they cash them out. One can also take money out when needed. For example, if in financial straits, or one can use the money to buy a house or get an education. However such withdrawals are taxable upon withdrawal regardless of the reason for doing so. This plan can be self-directed (i.e. one can make investments oneself) or it can be directed by financial experts who specialize in making investments. There are also Group RRSPs which involve a number of individual accounts set up through an employer generally as an alternative to on RPP.

RPP's is a particularly mystifying term, referring as it does to an employer-sponsored plan. RPP's are more commonly known as a workplace pension plans, private plans or occupational plans. RPP's are established on a voluntary basis, either by employers or unions in both the private and public sectors and their purpose is to provide retirement incomes to employees. Employers offering an RPP are required by law to contribute to it.

Legislative changes now allow part-time employees to be covered. RPP's may consist of either defined benefits or defined contributions. Employers are not compelled to establish such a plan. RRIF's refer to the requirement that the funds in RRSPs be withdrawn at age now seventy-one, taken as a taxable lump sum, or invested in an RRIF or an annuity. RRIF, funds must be withdrawn annually, based on actuarially defined amounts to ensure that the fund is empty by the time the contributor reaches age ninety. Taxes are paid on all these required withdrawals. Deferred profit-sharing plans offer another option, but few take it.

There are other factors concerning the three tiers, but the information just presented covers the basics. Further information is available through Human Resources Development Canada, Service Canada, on the Internet, from an accountant or by consulting a financial advisor. A number of community-based organizations may also be helpful.

Index

A

advocacy; advocates; 362-367, 373, 386, 391, 394, 362, 367, 368, 374

American Association of Retired Persons (AARP); 265

anti-aging; 138-140
   and internet; 183

advertisers, advertising; 86

ageism, ageist; 31

anorexia; 96-98

B

Butler, Robert; 19

C

Canada Pension Plan; 224-233 *cf. Appendix 2*

Canadian boomers; 19

Chappell, Neena; 262

Childcare; 264, 266, 289-287, 293

Clinton, Hillary; 35-37

Connidis, Ingrid; 270, 343

consciousness; 369, 384, 400-402

conservatism, neo-conservatism; 362, 367, 368, 374
consumer; 49
cosmetic surgery ; 103-105
Cruikshank, Margaret; 18

D

decline; 67
development; 17
disability; 159-164
divorce; 204
Dove soap; 103-105

E

earnings by gender; 20
Ehrenreich, Barbara and English, Deirdre; 131-133

F

film 59-67
fitness; 152-159
Friedan, Betty; 16
Furman, Frida ; 106

G

globalized; 91
great depression; 89
greeting cards; 53-57
Gullette, Margaret Morganroth; 18

H

Health care
  of separated, divorced; 177-178
health care system Canada; 153, 170-179
  privatization of; 170-179
home care; 216
hormone; 143-5
humor; 56
hysterical; 131-133

I

intergenerational 259
Internet, and anti-aging 83

K

Kemp, Candace; 264

L

language; 37-43
little girls; 95

M

marketing; 82
Mc Daniel, Susan; 212
McDonald, Lynn; 232
media, and sexism; 37-43
medicalization; 140
menopause, menopausal; 141-146
misogynist; 33
mother/daughter; 322-325

O

obesity; 157-158

P

parental leave; 214-215
pharmaceutical corporations; 134-141
physicians, health practitioners; 164-9
plastic surgery; 106-113
policy; 370-375
population aging; 15, 203

post-menopausal women; 34

R

Relationships as buffer; 318
resistance; 380-384
Rosenthal, Carolyn; 266

S

Schor, Juliet; 95
seniors; 42
sexist language; 12-13
  and media; 37-43
sexuality; 146-152
sexualization; 95-96
sisters, siblings; 342
stereotypes; 40
successful aging; 32
syndrome; 136-138

T

toddlers; 89
Townson, Monica; 201
TV, television; 43-53

U

unpaid work; 195, 197, 210-16, 218, 219, 220, 231

W

Wendell, Sue; 160-161
widowhood; 206
Wister, Andrew; 156-159
witches; 35
Wolf, Naomi; 88
women's movement; 69-70
workplace pensions; 227

Acknowledgements

To my friends and colleagues, many of whom are both, thank you for advice, critiques and encouragement in various degrees as needed (in no particular order):

Anita Fellman, Raymond Adams, Joanne Richardson, Melody Hessing, Fraidie Martz, Olive Johnson, Bonnie S.Klein, Susan Witter, Myrna Levy, Barbara Mitchell, Angela Johnston, Andrew Wister, Margaret Fulton, Susan McDaniel, Nita Joy, Michael Mills, Adrienne Chan, Monica Townson, Sandra Cusack, Gordon Gee, Ross Johnson, and Barbara Clague.

Narratives express the soul of women's experiences. I am deeply grateful to the women who attended the focus groups which I organized around this book's topics, for their spirit, generosity and openness in expressing their feelings.

To my multi-talented editor James Dangerous, for his editing skills, breadth of knowledge, and for being a communicator par excellence, thank you.

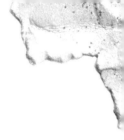
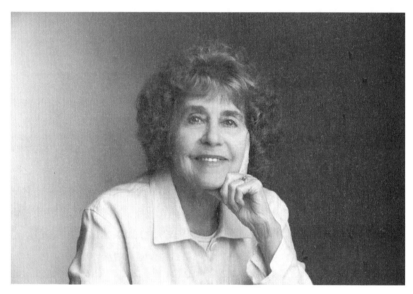

Lillian Zimmerman. Photo by Michael Mills.

About the Author

LILLIAN ZIMMERMAN, Research Associate, Gerontololgy Research Centre at Simon Fraser University, Vancouver, has a B.A. in Sociology from SFU and a Masters in Social Work, UBC. She is an Adult Educator, spending many years building and promoting the concept of Lifelong Learning. She was a faculty member at Douglas College, New Westminster B.C., latterly as Chair of the Department of Continuing and Community Education, and an early proponent of Women's Studies. Upon retirement, she started another career in Gerontology with a particular interest in policies related to men, such as work, retirement, pensions, and intergenerational issues. She has written, lectured, presented at national conferences and organized conferences on these topics. Throughout her professional career and personal life, Zimmerman's prime interest has always been perspectives of women. She now tops this lifelong work with this innovative and powerful book.